Contents

Introduction

Urology, arguably the oldest speciality, has now assumed its rightful place in the forefront of surgical practice, as it embraces 30 per cent of all surgical problems. As in the last two decades significant progress has been made in all branches of urology, it can no longer be considered within the precincts of the general surgeon, although until further expansion of urological appointments has taken place, it is accepted that many urological cases will have to be treated by general surgeons throughout the world.

This book is therefore aimed at a comprehensive readership embracing senior clinical students, junior urologists at all stages of their training and general surgeons with an interest in urology. It is hoped also that the practising urologist will find something of value, because we have attempted to include many of the results of the exciting scientific advances which have taken place in urology in recent years.

Much of the information is basic; for this we make no apology, because we consider it is fundamental to have a sound knowledge of first principles.

Successful diagnosis is based on a combination of clinical acumen and the interpretation of appropriate investigations. We have combined investigations, macropathology and histopathology with normal and special stains and where appropriate endoscopic photography to emphasise the importance of inter-disciplinary co-operation in urology.

The first chapter is therefore a description of standard urological investigations, together with tables of normal values which can be used as a reference to compare results obtained in various pathological conditions.

In recent years urodynamics has begun to play an ever-increasing role in the investigation of disorders of micturition; consequently this diagnostic procedure has been included in some detail.

The discovery of Professor Hopkins of the rod lens system and the flexible glass fibre bundles has revolutionised endoscopy. It is now possible to portray with sufficient detail and accurate colour rendering, lesions in the urethra and bladder. A considerable part of this book has been devoted to this aspect of urology, so that endoscopists can become more readily acquainted with the normal and abnormal appearances of the urethra and bladder.

The boundary between urology and nephrology is often obscure and deceptive and we are conscious that we may have trespassed into their territory. However, we feel that if a true understanding is to be achieved it is impossible not to invade the ground more properly assigned to them, and if in doing so we have made unacceptable errors we ask for their understanding.

In this book we have attempted to include as many as possible of the commoner conditions and some of the rare diseases. It is not meant, however, to compete with textbooks of urology but to complement them and to be appreciated as a pictorial record encompassing a broad spectrum of urology.

We have not sought in any way to cover paediatric urology and have made only brief mention of renal failure and venereology and trauma, because we considered they were not subjects suitable to this kind of presentation.

Because it is an atlas the introductory texts and legends are short and are used only to highlight the more important points of each illustration.

We hope that it will be treated not just as a reference but will act as a stimulus to provoke the reader to delve deeper into the many exciting projects which have now become part of the practice of urology.

In such a book there will be many omissions particularly among the rarer diseases; for this we can only crave the indulgence of the reader and hope that it may be possible to correct them in subsequent editions.

Acknowledgements

We are very grateful to our colleagues, without whose help and encouragement this Atlas could not have been completed. Mr K.E.D. Shuttleworth, Mr N.O.K. Gibbon, Mr R.M. Jamieson and Mr M.R. Heal have contributed a large range of Diagnostic problems, and Mr M.I. Bultitude has been particularly helpful with the section on Urodynamics. Dr A. Carty, Dr N.H. Crosby, Dr J.H.E. Carmichael, Dr A.B. Ayers, Dr M. Lea-Thomas and Dr J. Pemberton, our Radiological colleagues, have been very helpful, and to them we are most appreciative.

Dr A.B. Ayers in addition has given a notable contribution to the ultrasound studies. Dr E.W. Lupton has been most generous in supplying the Renograms, and we are very indebted to him. We also thank Mr W.B. Peeling and his colleagues Mr P.J. Brooman, Dr G.H. Griffiths, Dr K.T. Evans and Mr E.E. Roberts for their help with the new technique of prostatic imaging by perirectal ultrasonography. Brunel and Kjaer (UK) Ltd., have generously donated slides **821**, **821a** and **821b**, illustrating the latest technique for intravesical ultrasonography. Mr F.T. Graves has been very kind in allowing us to use photographs **50**, **51**, **52a**, **52b**, **121a** and **144b**, which are reproduced by permission of John Wright & Son, Bristol and F.T. Graves in whose monograph *The Arterial Anatomy of the Kidney, the basis of Surgical Technique* further details of the intrarenal vascular system can be found.

We wish to thank the many colleagues listed below for the loan of illustrations. Dr A.B. Ayers (**26**, **27**, **27a**, **28**, **28a**, **156**, **189a** and **b**, **190a** and **b**, **651a** and **b**, **652a** and **b**, **700a** and **b**, **701a** and **b**); Dr M. Black and his colleagues of The Department of Dermatology, St Thomas' Hospital· (**1090**, **1091**); Mr N. Blackford; Dr Blackwell (**1033**, **1034**); Mr M.I. Bultitude (**95** to **107**); Dr R.D. Catterall (**971**); Mr P.B. Clark (**317**, **853**); Dr C.D. Collins (**1138**, **1139**); Mr D. Davies for the TB preparations from which **348** to **351** were taken; Professor El Ghorab and Dr N. Badr for providing most of the non-histological Bilharzia slides; Mr R. Ewing (**1018**); Dr S. Eykyn (**66**, **67**, **68**); Mr C. Gingell (**987**, **1025**, **1046**, **1054** to **1065**, **1070**, **1074**, **1075**, **1084**, **1086**, **1115**, **1116**, **1119**, **1127**, **1128**); Mr W.F. Hendry (**1122**, **1124**); Dr Eadie Heyderman for the histology sections from which **1154** and **1168** were taken; Mr J.P. Hopewell (**1029**); Professor M.S.R. Hutt (**478**), and for allowing us access to his collection of tropical pathological slides; Dr N.F. Jones (**757** to **758**); Mr C.H. Kinder (**281**); Professor J.B. Kinmonth (**341**, **342**); Dr D. Lowe (**971**); Dr C. Parkinson for the sections from which **773**, **774**, **854** and **855** were taken; Dr C. Pike for the cytology preparation from which **776** and **777** were taken; Mr W.B. Peeling and his colleagues (**29**, **30**, **31a** and **b**, **32a** and **b**, **82a** and **b**, **863**, **864**, **935** to **940**, **1134** to **1137**); Dr J. Pincott (**157a**); Mr J.M. Pullan (**1142**); The Royal Tropical Institute (**454** to **459**); Professor J.B. Stewart (**1165**); Mr T.A. Taylor (**1025**); Dr K. Thomas (**1173**); Professor J.R. Tighe (**334**) and for allowing us access to the files of the Histopathology Department, St Thomas' Hospital; Dr Lyal Walker (**506**); and Mr R.H. Whitaker (**47** to **49** and **185** to **188**).

histology slides; Mr V. Clarke for the photography of many of the pathological specimens; Mr T. Brandon and his staff, Photographic Department, St Thomas' Hospital; Mr W.C. Fitzsimmons and his staff, Photographic Department, Liverpool Eastern District and Mr J. Stammers and his staff, Central Photographic Department, University of Liverpool. Mr Ken Biggs, Medical Artist, Anatomy Department, University of Liverpool has been responsible for the line drawings and the excellent colour diagrams, and his superb technique has added considerable distinction to the Atlas.

No work such as this could be completed without the help and sympathetic understanding of our secretaries, Mrs J.E. Stephens, Mrs N.M. Williams, Mrs B.D. Worthington and Miss M. Murphy, and to them we shall always be most grateful.

1   Investigations

In the management of any urological patient there are three main facets. First and most important is the history, second is the clinical examination and third there are the ancillary investigations which are considered appropriate to the clinical assessment.

Radiology

Intravenous urogram (IVU)

The excretory urogram demonstrates anatomical features of the renal substance and the pelvicalyceal system, and at the same time gives some information about the functional capacity of the whole system. There are two phases: first the nephrogram which outlines the upper nephron as most of the water reabsorption takes place in the proximal tubules. This phase demonstrates functional renal tissue and so the density of the nephrogram is important as it will help in assessing the quality of glomerular filtration.

1   Dense nephrogram indicating good glomerular filtration.

2   Paler nephrogram suggesting some impairment of glomerular function.

The second phase is to outline the calyces, pelvis and ureters which depend on water reabsorption and hence the level of hydration of the patient.

3   Normal intravenous urogram.

4   An oblique view of a normal upper urinary tract which often helps to outline a small calyceal lesion.

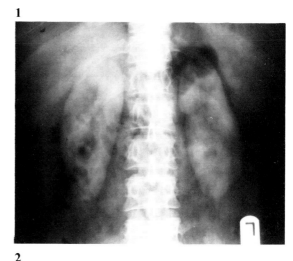

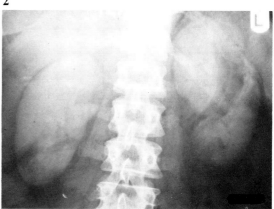

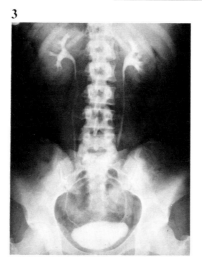

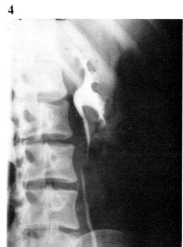

5 IVU normal cystogram in which the bladder outline is smooth and regular.

6 IVU normal post-micturition film in which the dye is seen between the folds of the flaccid mucus membrane.

5

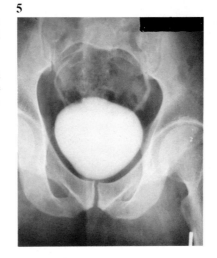

6

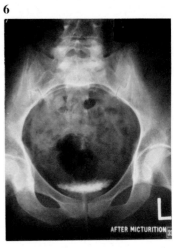

7a

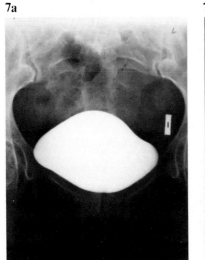

7b

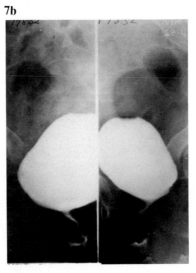

7c

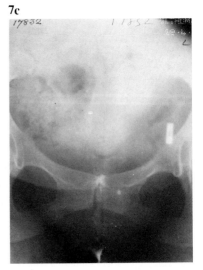

7a, b and c Normal micturating cystourethrogram in the female: a) full bladder; b) during micturition (oblique views to show reflux if present); c) after micturition.

8

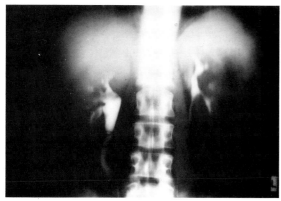

9

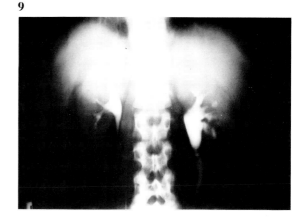

10

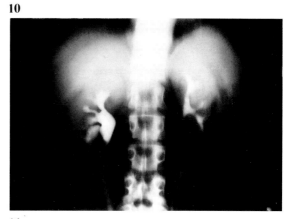

Tomograms are useful adjuncts to the conventional urogram in helping to differentiate whether a lesion is in the anterior, middle or posterior part of the kidney, especially in the presence of intestinal gas.

8   **Tomogram of both kidneys** with 5 cm cut.

9   **Tomogram of both kidneys** with 6 cm cut.

10   **Tomogram of both kidneys** with 7 cm cut.

Pyelovenous backflow

What was originally thought to be pyelovenous backflow is now (with modern high-dose techniques) considered to be a concentration of dye in the collecting tubules giving a dense pyramidal outline.

11   **Diffuse pyramidal contrast.**

11

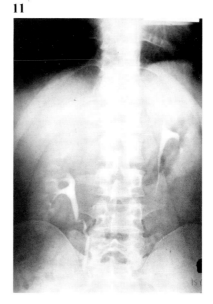

12   Catheter in a ureteric orifice.

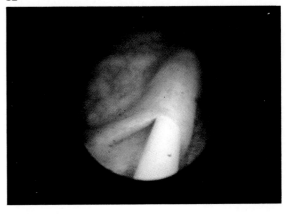

Retrograde pyelography

This procedure is used less frequently as a result of the improved pictures produced by the intravenous urogram. When retrograde pyelography is required it should first be performed through a bulb catheter, so that a dynamic study of the ureter can be carried out, using the image intensifier at the time of the injection. Later, a catheter can, if required, be passed to the kidney.

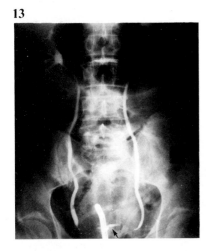

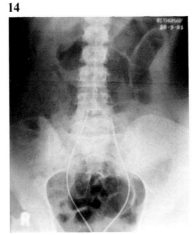

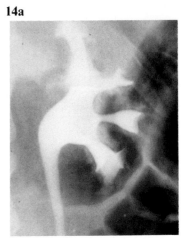

13   Bilateral normal retrograde ureterogram. Note bulb-ended catheter.

14   Bilateral retrograde catheters in situ.

14a   Fine detail of pelvicalyceal system.

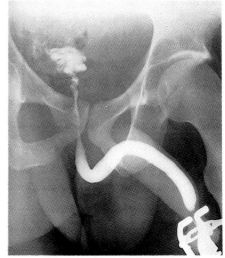

15   Normal ascending urethrogram. The urethra is smooth and always becomes narrow in the region of the external sphincter. The verumontanum is shown as a filling defect in the prostatic urethra.

Arteriography

Selective renal arteriography is usually carried out by passing a catheter up the femoral artery and guiding it into the renal artery under direct vision. If this method is not possible, either the axillary artery or a translumbar aortic puncture may be used.

The arteriogram is carried out in four phases.

16 Flush arteriogram, which shows the vascular tree and architecture, of both kidneys, and will identify plaques in the renal artery.

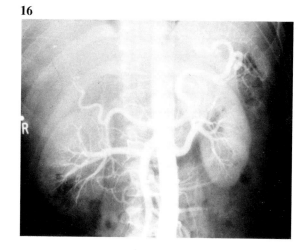

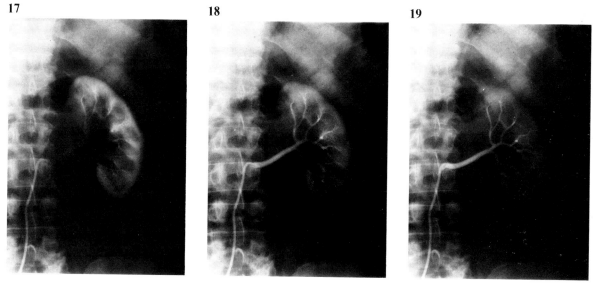

17 Nephrographic phase, which demonstrates the small vessels in the cortex.

18 and 19 Early and late vascular phases, when the main vessels become more obvious.

20

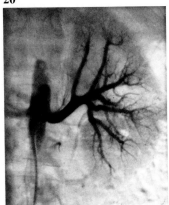

21

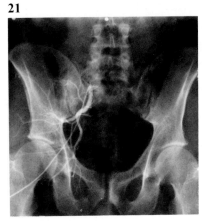

22

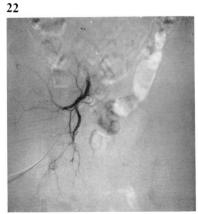

Subtraction arteriogram

A subtraction arteriogram is useful in assessing the vascular flush of malignant renal tumours, because it highlights the vessels in much greater detail.

20 Normal subtraction renal arteriogram.

21 and 22 Arteriogram and subtraction arteriogram of the internal iliac artery showing up the pudendal artery. An essential investigation in some cases of impotence.

Inferior venocavogram

A cavogram may be important in assessing the spread of lesions such as a renal carcinoma, because it will show renal vein obstruction.

23 Normal subtraction cavogram.

23

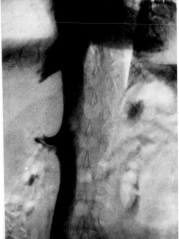

Lymphography

Abdominal lymphography is used as a guide in the staging of various malignant conditions, such as testicular tumours and carcinoma of the prostate. It is indicated in investigating patients with lymph node enlargement of obscure cause, chyluria, lymphoma, retroperitoneal fibrosis, testicular tumours, carcinoma of the prostate, and carcinoma of the penis.

24 Normal lymphogram. Lymphadenogram phase showing normal nodes.

24

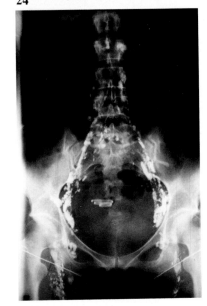

Seminal vesiculogram

A seminal vesiculogram is an occasional investigation carried out to exclude obstructive lesions in the ejaculatory system, especially those close to the verumontanum.

25 Normal vesiculogram.

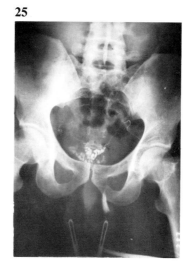

25

Computerised axial tomography (CAT)

Computerised axial tomography is the reconstruction by a computer of a radiographic tomographic image through a particular plane of the body. This procedure is used with intravenous urography to study renal pathology.

26 and 26a Normal cat scan at the level of D^{12} showing both kidneys, aorta, inferior vena cava and abdominal contents.

26

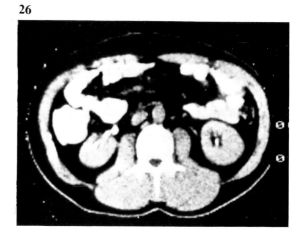

26a

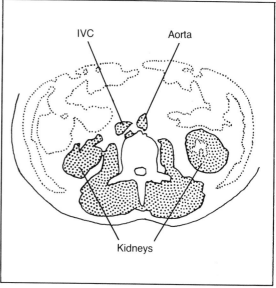

IVC Aorta

Kidneys

27

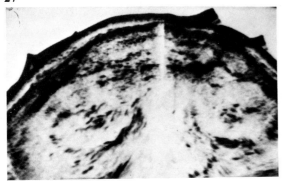

27a

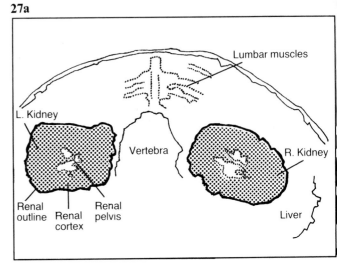

Ultrasound

Ultrasound is a non-invasive technique based on sonography. It does not require the injection of contrast media when it is used to evaluate cystic and solid renal masses or to localise accurately needles for aspiration, biopsy or percutaneous nephrostomy.

27 and 27a   Normal transverse ultrasound of renal area.

28

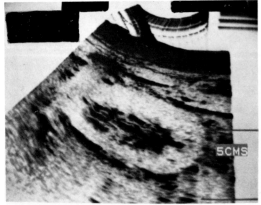

28a

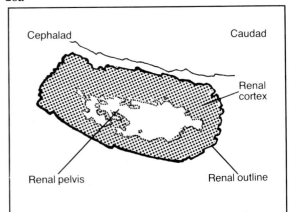

28 and 28a   Normal longitudinal ultrasound of renal area.

This technique can also be used in the investigation of prostatic lesions.

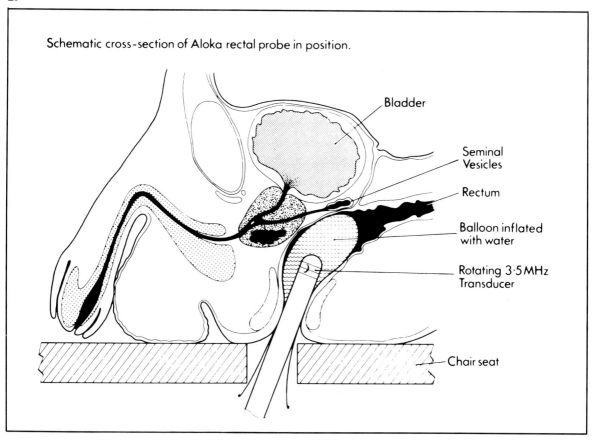

Schematic cross-section of Aloka rectal probe in position.

Bladder

Seminal Vesicles

Rectum

Balloon inflated with water

Rotating 3·5 MHz Transducer

Chair seat

Prostatic imaging by per-rectal ultrasonography

The diagnosis of prostatic disease by rectal palpation is notoriously inaccurate, especially for the smaller nodule and only the back and posterolateral parts of the gland are accessible to palpation and thus to needle biopsy.

Imaging of the prostate aims to give an objective record of the whole prostate gland and demonstrates the prostatic capsule at all levels, the seminal vesicles and bladder base, and differentiates abnormal from normal tissues, also allowing measurement of prostatic dimensions.

The prostate is imaged with an ultrasound probe with a rotating transducer mounted on a chair and introduced through the anal canal so that it just enters the lower rectum.

29 A water-filled balloon surrounds the probe tip and the transducer rotates radially to give 360° scans of the pelvis, and by withdrawal of the probe at 0.5 cm intervals, ultrasonograms of the prostate from the bladder base and seminal vesicles to the prostatic apex can be obtained.

30

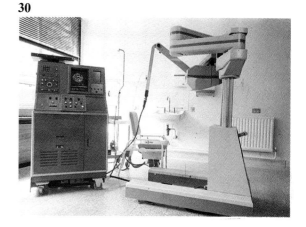

30 The probe is linked to a Grayscale scanner incorporating a digital scan converter and micro-processor to improve image resolution. The image is displayed on a screen and photographed.

An electronic cursor outlining the prostatic capsule allows volume measurements of the prostate.

31a

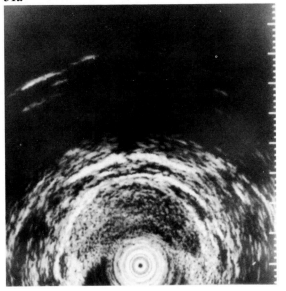

31b

Right   Left

Prostatic
capsule

Pelvic
tissues

Probe in rectum

Normal features

31a and b Scan and explanatory diagram of normal prostate showing a crescent-shaped capsule that is intact at all levels of scanning, with, in general, a homogenous echo pattern of the parenchyma. Complete homogeneity of parenchyma is rare. The urethra is rarely identified.

32a and b Scan and explanatory diagram of seminal vesicles (SV) which appear as transonic curved zones behind the base of the bladder.

32a

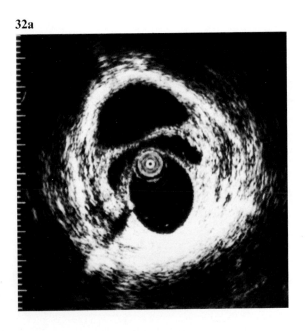

32b

Right   Left

Bladder

S.V.

S.V.

Rectum

Cyst puncture

Cyst puncture is now a normal method of investigating not only the outline of cysts, but also for making a detailed examination of the cyst contents.

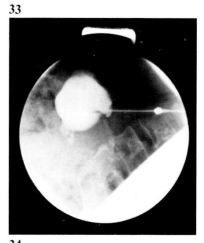

33 Normal cyst puncture. This technique is particularly useful in the diagnosis of cystic renal lesions.

Renal biopsy

A renal biopsy may be the only way to make the exact diagnosis, but it is not without its hazards and should not be lightly undertaken.

34 Arteriovenous fistula after renal biopsy.

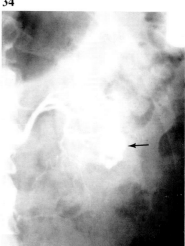

Renal scan

Using scintillation counters over each kidney after the intravenous injection of an isotope compound, the concentration of this compound will give an accurate assessment of the function of each kidney. The examination is carried out in two parts – parenchymal and vascular – the parenchymal studying renal function and the vascular renal perfusion, which especially detects areas of greater or lesser vascularity. The whole investigation is a combination of an angiogram and nephrogram.

Radioisotope renal scans

With the development of the gamma-camera linked to a mini-computer, renal scintigraphy has been increasingly used in the investigation of the urinary tract. Two types of scan are in widespread use – the Static scan using $^{99}Tc^m$-DMSA (Dimercaptosuccinnic acid) and the Dynamic scan using $^{99}Tc^m$-DTPA (Diethylenetriamine pentacetic acid). I^{123} sodium iodohippurate has also been used extensively for this purpose.

Static scans are useful in the detection and quantitation of functioning renal cortical tissue. The main use of static scans is in the assessment of differential renal function but they have also been used in the investigation of renal tumours.

In dynamic scans the passage of the labelled DTPA through the urinary tract is recorded on serial 'frames' for 20 to 30 minutes after the intravenous injection of a bolus of $^{99}Tc^m$-DTPA. Subsequently background – subtracted Time-Activity curves may be derived for each kidney (or part of kidney) and the bladder. Analysis of these curves allows the clinician to comment on the vascularity, cortical function and the drainage of the urine from the kidney. Thus dynamic scans are useful in the assessment of renal failure, renal vascular disease, renal outflow obstruction, vesicoureteric reflux and, especially, renal transplantation.

Radioisotope renal scans in no way replace the IVU as an investigative procedure. However, they provide much additional information regarding the function of the kidneys, much of which could only otherwise be obtained by more invasive techniques.

35 Normal gamma camera sodium iodiohippurate 2 minutes after injection of I^{123} sodium iodohippurate.

36 Normal parenchymal study 3 to 5 minutes after injection of 99MTc.

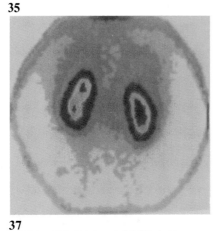
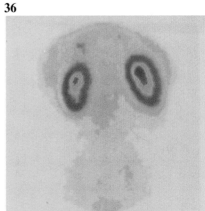

37 Normal gamma camera sodium iodohippurate 8 minutes after injection of I^{123} sodium iodohippurate.

38 Normal gamma camera sodium iodohippurate 12 minutes after injection of I^{123} sodium iodohippurate.

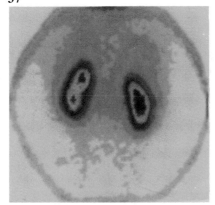
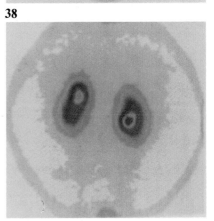

39 Normal gamma camera sodium iodohippurate 17 minutes after injection of I^{123} sodium iodohippurate.

40 Normal gamma camera sodium iodohippurate 25 minutes after injection of I^{123} sodium iodohippurate.

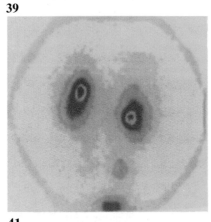
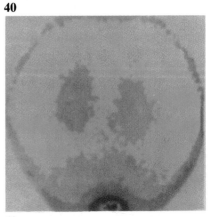

41 Normal vascularity 15 to 20 seconds after 99HH^c radiophane centica.

42 Normal combined vascular and parenchymatous phase.

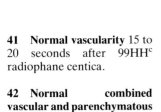
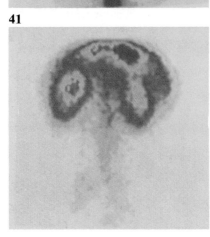
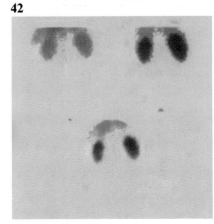

43

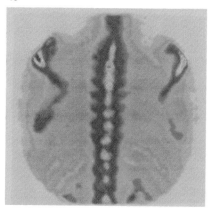

Bone scan

Bone scanning involves bone minerals reacting with specific agents. The commonest are 99^{M}Tc-labelled phosphorus containing compounds. The images which are produced are recorded by a scanning gamma camera.

43 Normal appearance of the bone scan of the chest and abdominal cavity.

44a and b Bone scan showing normal uptake in the skull, clavicle, cervical upper dorsal spine and pelvis.

44a

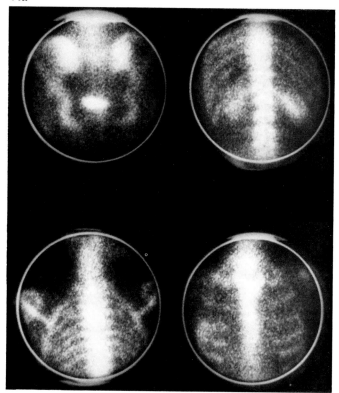

44b

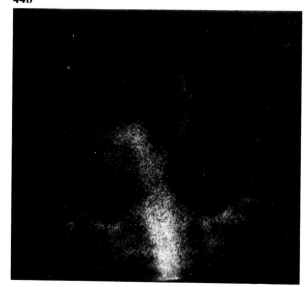

45

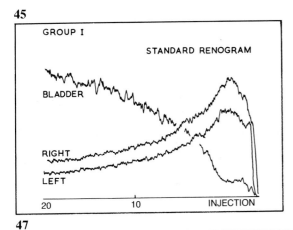

GROUP I

STANDARD RENOGRAM

BLADDER

RIGHT

LEFT

20   10   INJECTION

46

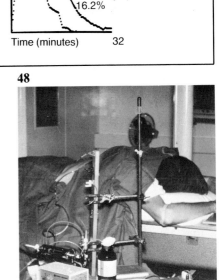

23%

Max uptake lt kidney 21.6%

Max uptake rt kidney 22.2%

Lt kidney uptake at 3 minutes 18.9%

Rt kidney uptake at 3 minutes 16.2%

Time (minutes)   32

47

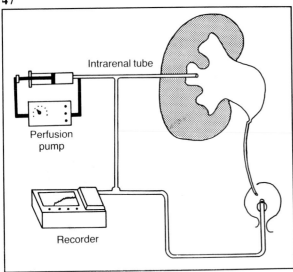

Intrarenal tube

Perfusion pump

Recorder

48

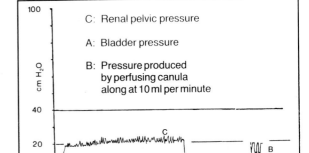

49

100

C: Renal pelvic pressure

A: Bladder pressure

B: Pressure produced by perfusing canula along at 10 ml per minute

cm H_2O

40

20

C

0

A

B

Time: minutes

Renograms

45   Normal renogram. Three phases occur: 1 Isotope arriving in the renal artery; 2 Intrarenal transit time; 3 Shows disappearance of the isotope from the upper urinary tract.

During the second and third phases a bladder accumulation curve develops.

Diuresis renogram

The diuresis renogram is a modification of the routine renogram and is helpful in differentiating between a hypotonic and obstructive hydronephrosis.

46   Diuresis renogram: normal standard on the right side. Note the rapid fall on the left side after the diuretic has been injected, indicating no obstruction at the pelvi-ureteric junction.

The Whitaker test

The apparatus measures the pressure drop between the renal pelvis and the bladder and is another method of differentiating between an obstructive or non-obstructive lesion in the urinary tract. A pressure drop of less than 10 cm of water at an injection rate of 10 ml per minute indicates no obstruction.

47   Diagram of apparatus for investigating a pelvi-ureteric obstruction. Pressure is measured in the pelvis and the bladder at a perfusion of 10 ml per minute.

48   Apparatus in use showing position of the patient, renal cannula in position, perfusion pump and recorder.

49   Normal recording.

50

51

52a

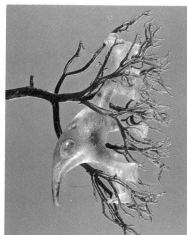

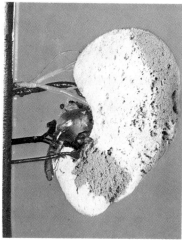

52b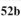

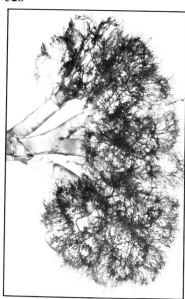

52c

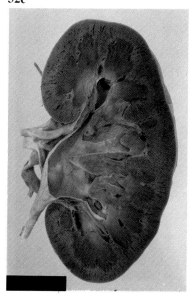

Blood supply of normal kidney

50   Blood supply cast. The main stem of the renal artery divides into an anterior and posterior division; the anterior division supplies four segments on the front of the kidney – the apical segment, the upper segment, the middle segment and the lower segment. The posterior division continues into and becomes the artery to the posterior segment, which occupies a large central area on the back of the organ. In this cast, the divisions are so short that the anterior division of the renal artery divides into its segmental branches almost at one point.

51   Posterior view of the same cast of the right kidney. The posterior division arises from the main stem of the renal artery to supply two-thirds of the renal substance on the posterior aspect of the organ. As it approaches the hilum, it becomes continuous with the artery of the posterior segment, which in turn divides into three sets of branches – an upper, a middle and a terminal group. The area supplied by the last (and lowest) of these three vessels is adjacent to, and above, the territory of the posterior branch of the lower segment artery. (Branch of the anterior division.)

52a   Renal arterial supply by multiple vessels. Some kidneys are supplied by multiple arteries. This cast shows a kidney seen from behind, supplied by three segmental arteries, each of which has arisen directly from the aorta. Each artery was injected with a resin of a different colour. The apical segmental and the posterior segmental arteries are in yellow resin, which has become off-white because of the colour dilution in the finer vessels of the cortex. The anterior division supplying the upper and middle segments is in red resin. The anterior branch of the lower segment artery is in blue, and the posterior branch of the lower segment artery is in red resin.

52b   Cast of the venous drainage of a normal kidney.

52c   Normal kidney. A bisected normal kidney showing capsule, cortex, medulla, pelvis and ureter, pelvic fat and vessels at the hilum (formalin fixed).

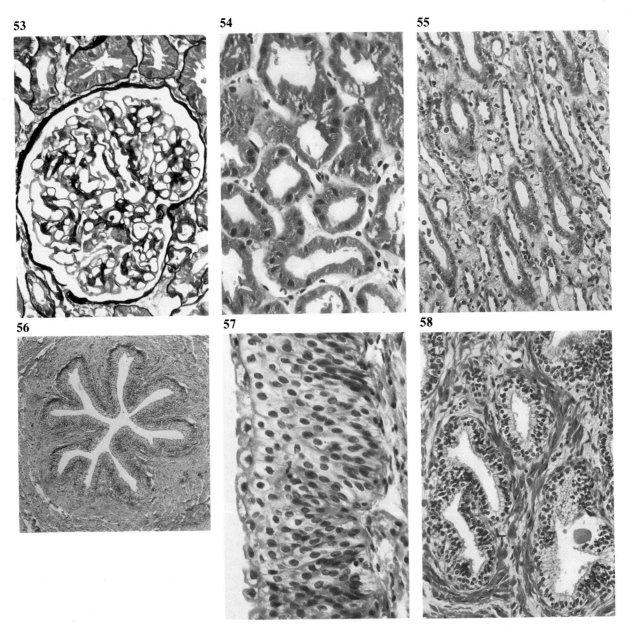

53

54

55

56

57

58

55 Kidney: medullary tubules. The collecting tubules and the loops of Henle are seen in the medulla. *(H&E × 160)*

53 Normal glomerulus: section through a glomerulus showing the hilum at the right of the field. Bowman's capsule surrounds the urinary space within which is the glomerular tuft. This is made up of capillaries communicating with the afferent and efferent arterioles at the hilum. In the tuft the methenamine silver picks up the basement membrane and mesangial matrix. The capillaries are open and the urinary filtrate is formed across the basement membrane (with its endothelial and epithelial cells) into the urinary space. *(Methenamine silver × 256)*

54 Kidney: cortical tubules. The proximal and distal convoluted tubules are situated in the cortex and modify the glomerular filtrate. *(H&E × 256)*

56 Ureter. The ureter is lined with transitional epithelium. A little subepithelial connective tissue is present and then the muscle coats. There is an inner longitudinal layer and an outer circular layer with a second longitudinal layer in the lower third. The adventitia is outside the muscle. *(H&E × 26)*

57 Transitional epithelium lines the urothelial tract from the renal pelvis to the urethra. It is a multilayered epithelium, normally up to about seven layers thick. The most superficial cells are wider and cover a few underlying cells. This section is from a ureter. *(H&E × 256)*

58 Prostate. Normal prostatic glands in fibromuscular stroma. *(H&E × 160)*

59 **Prostate showing normal-size lobes and urethra** from a 24-year-old male dying from unrelated lesions.

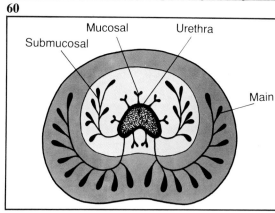

60 **Diagram of duct system of the lobes of the prostate.**

Mucosal · Urethra · Submucosal · Main

61 **Urethra and verumontanum.** Prostatic ducts opening on verumontanum into the urethra on the right of the field. *(H&E × 64)*

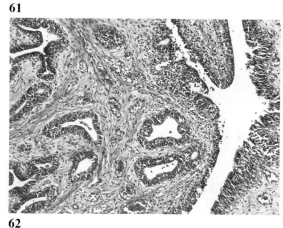

62 **Vas deferens.** This duct is lined by columnar, pseudostratified epithelium and surrounded by three muscle coats, an inner and an outer longitudinal and a middle circular layer. *(H&E × 16)*

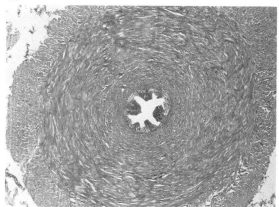

63 Testis and epididymis. Testicular tubules on right-hand side of the field; epididymal tubules on the left.

The testis is a compound tubular gland divided into over 200 components, surrounded by a fibrous capsule, the tunica albuginea. They consist of seminiferous tubules which show spermatogenesis with spermatozoa in various stages of maturation, Sertoli cells which are attached to the basement membrane are also seen. The interstitial tissue consists of connective tissue, blood and lymph vessels, a few cells and the cells of Leydig. (See also **1182** and **1183**.)

The seminiferous tubules pass into the rete testis and form the ducti efferentes, which pass through the head, body and tail of the epididymis to form the vas deferens. In the proximal part of the epididymis the lumen is lined by pseudostratified columnar epithelium, but the cells disappear as the ductus epididymis approaches the globus minor.

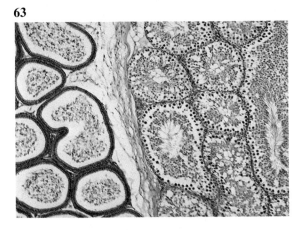

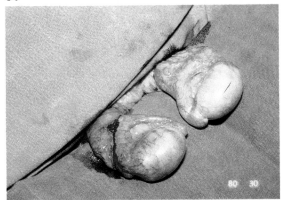

64 Testes and epididymes.

65 Diagram of testis and duct system.

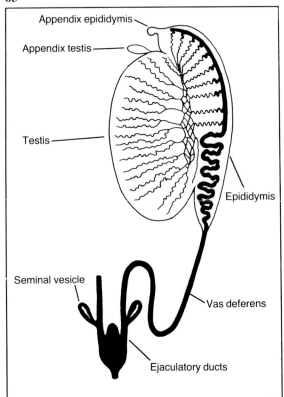

Appendix epididymis

Appendix testis

Testis

Epididymis

Seminal vesicle

Vas deferens

Ejaculatory ducts

Crystals

Amorphous phosphates Fine granular forms, often found in urine which has been standing for some time and may be mistaken for bacteria by the inexperienced microscopist.

Calcium oxalate 'envelope' crystals.

Triple phosphates (Ammonium magnesium phosphate) 'coffin-lid' crystals of varying size.

66, 67 and 68   Crystals in the urine: 66 Amorphous phosphates; **67** Calcium oxalate; **68** Triple phosphate.

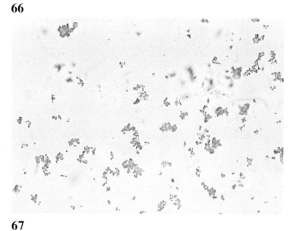

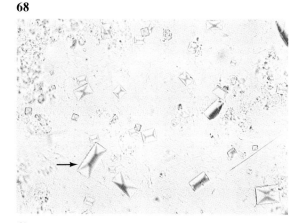

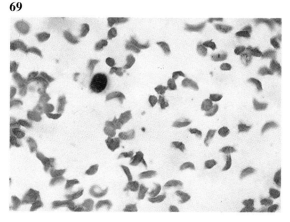

Haematology

Sickle-cell disease. Haemoglobinopathy is seen in negroid races. The abnormality is that one amino-acid, glutamic acid, is substituted by valine in the sixth position of the amino-acid chain of haemoglobin. This alters the solubility of haemoglobin under reduced oxygen tension causing it to become less soluble and to crystallise out, producing the classical sickle shaped red cells, shown in **69**, which may lead to haematurin and produce renal lesions.

70

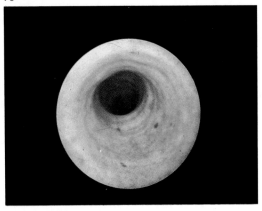

71

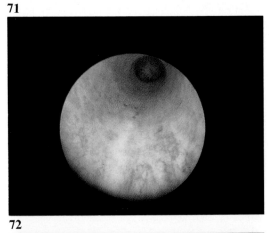

72

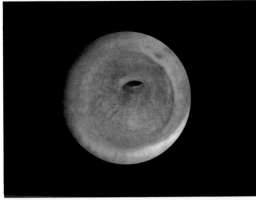

73

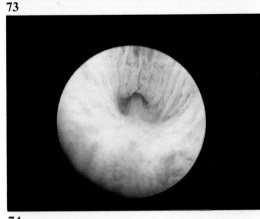

74

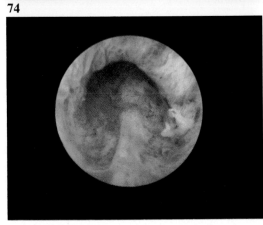

Endoscopy

70 Anterior urethra showing vascular pattern which in this part of the urethra is irregular.

71 Bulbous urethra showing change in the vascular pattern, a greater number of vessels are present and they are conforming to a more longitudinal arrangement.

72 Membranous urethra. The vessels now run longitudinally and converge towards the external sphincter.

73 External sphincter. The circular pattern is clearly seen. In the prostatic urethra there is a median ridge called the urethral crest, which extends from the bladder neck to the external sphincter. It is caused by an elevation of the mucus membrane and the underlying tissue. In the middle of the crest is the colliculus seminalis or verumontanum, on the tip of which open the ejaculatory ducts. On either side of the crest there is a depression into which the prostatic ducts open.

74 A normal urethral crest.

75

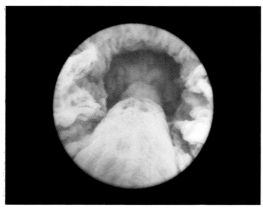

76

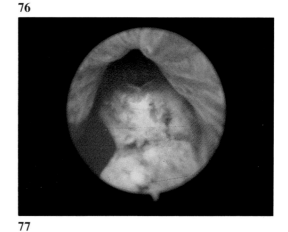

75 Verumontanum with the opening of the ejaculatory ducts clearly visible on the dome.

76 Lobulated verumontanum. A variant of the normal, but one which is liable to give rise to terminal haematuria.

77

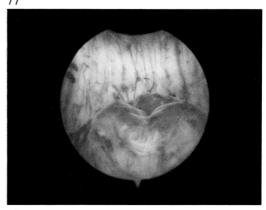

77 A more pronounced lobulation of the verumontanum.

78

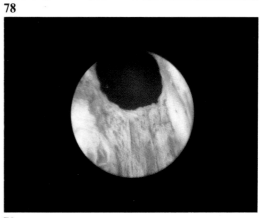

78 Normal bladder neck in a young male. The margins are smooth with a pronounced vascular pattern.

79

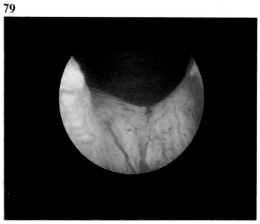

79 Normal bladder neck in a middle-aged male. The margins may be irregular and slight enlargement of the right lateral lobe of the prostate is visible.

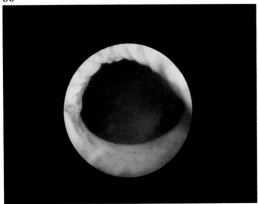

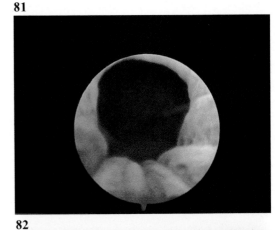

80 Normal bladder neck in a young female. The outline is smooth and merges posteriorly into the base of the bladder.

81 Normal bladder neck in a postmenopausal female. The mucus membrane is oedematous, more vascular and arranged in folds.

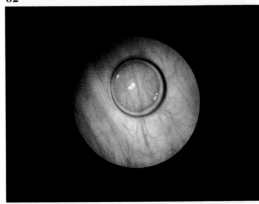

82 Air bubble, at the bladder fundus. An excellent initial landmark for the inexperienced urologist.

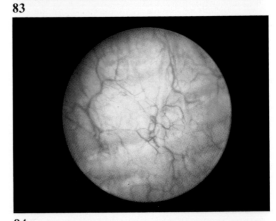

83 Normal bladder vessels.

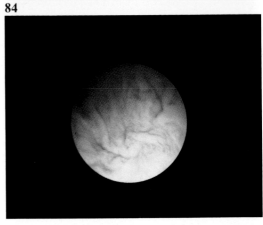

84 Flaccid mucus membrane. The normal appearance of the bladder before it is distended with fluid.

85

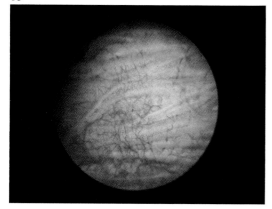

86

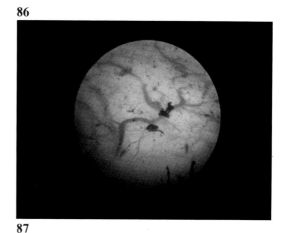

87

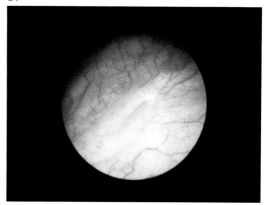

88

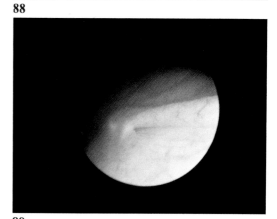

89

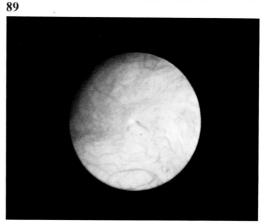

85 Normal bladder muscle. There is no set pattern. The individual muscle bundles appear as discrete strands which can be distinctly separated from each other.

86 Dilated bladder veins with petechial haemorrhages.

Variations of normal ureteric orifice

The final stages of development of the ureteric orifices are complex. The connection between the ureter and the bladder is brought about through Waldeyer's muscle sheath, which has a lateral and medial component both of which separate in the bladder to form different parts of the trigone. Therefore, it is not surprising that the normal ureteric orifice shows many variations.

87 The slit type of orifice.

88 Orifice on outer side of ureteric bar.

89 Shallow orifice with no ureteric bar.

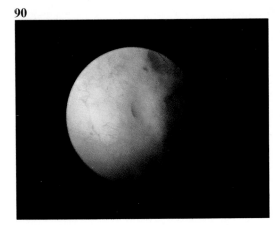

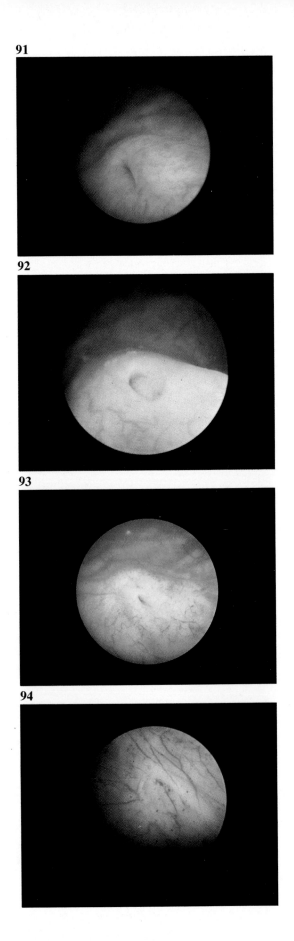

90 Orifice on top of a mound.

91 Stadium orifice.

92 Flat crescentic orifice.

93 Orifice with mild trabeculation.

94 Orifice which appears withdrawn and contracted.

Urodynamics

Cinecystometrogram

The patient is catheterised with either a double-lumen catheter or two catheters, the larger, through which the bladder is filled, is removed before micturition, the smaller measures bladder pressure. A further catheter in the rectum monitors abdominal pressure and can be subtracted from bladder pressure to give the true (intrinsic) bladder pressure. Males stand at and females sit on a commode beneath which a flow meter monitors the volume of urine passed and automatically computes the flow rate in millilitres per second (**95**). All parameters are recorded on a multichannel recorder and the chart viewed with a TV camera (**96**). The bladder is filled with radio-opaque fluid and viewed with an xray unit mounted on a 'C' arm for mobility (**97**). A split TV screen shows synchronously the measured parameters and cystogram image, and can be recorded on videotape. EMG of the external sphincters can also be recorded.

95 Male patient undergoing pressure-flow studies.

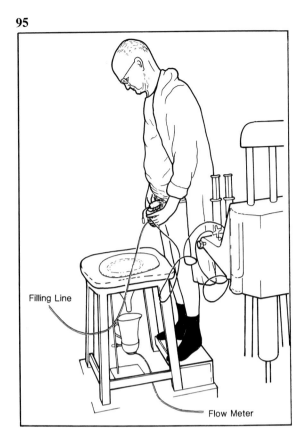

Filling Line

Flow Meter

96 Diagram of urodynamic apparatus.

96

MIXER BOX

FILLING PUMP

T.V. CAMERA

X RAY IMAGE INTENSIFIER

MONITOR

Rectal Pressure
Bladder Pressure
Intrinsil Pressure
Flow Volume

CHART RECORDER

VIDEO RECORDER

97 Male patient prepared for cinecystometrogram with image intensifier in place.

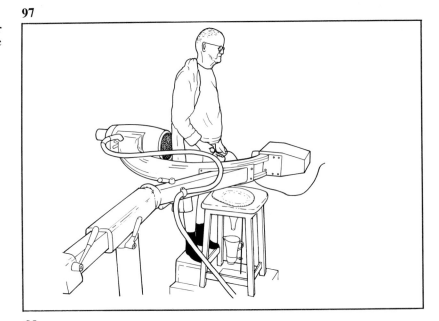

97

98 Urethral pressure profile equipment. A special catheter with a closed end and a rosette of subterminal openings is placed in the bladder. Fluid is slowly infused by means of a constant flow pump. The catheter is mechanically withdrawn at a constant rate and the pressure within the catheter recorded and, a profile of the static pressure conditions along the length of the urethra obtained. The patient can also be asked to contract the external sphincter and the alteration in the profile observed.

98

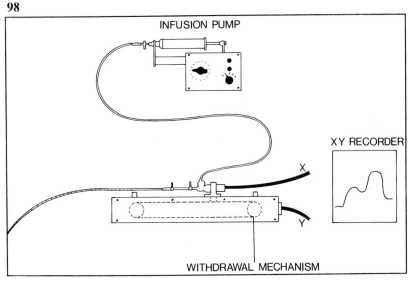

INFUSION PUMP

X Y RECORDER

X

Y

WITHDRAWAL MECHANISM

99

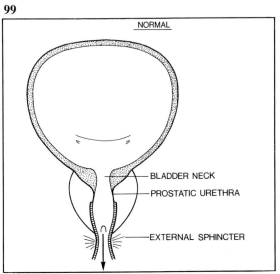

NORMAL

BLADDER NECK

PROSTATIC URETHRA

EXTERNAL SPHINCTER

99 Normal male bladder and urethra during micturition.

100 Pressure-flow study of normal micturition. In the normal bladder, filling results in a small pressure rise to the point of fullness. Micturition is under voluntary control and accomplished by a smooth increase in intravesical pressure as the detrusor contracts. Because detrusor fibres are inserted in the proximal urethra, the bladder neck is pulled open. The external sphincter coincidentally relaxes.

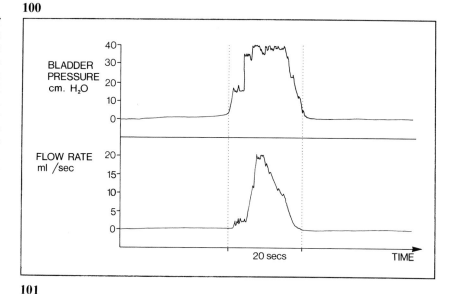

101 Pressure-flow study of detrusor instability. Involuntary uninhibited detrusor contractions occur as a result of overt neurological disease, representing an upper-motor neurone lesion, or may be seen as an idiopathic phenomenon. These contractions can cause frequency, urgency or frank incontinence. Alternatively, lower-motor neurone lesions result in low pressure 'autonomic' detrusor contractions and ineffective bladder emptying.

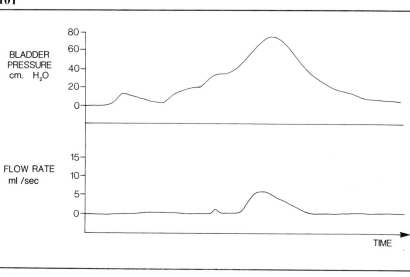

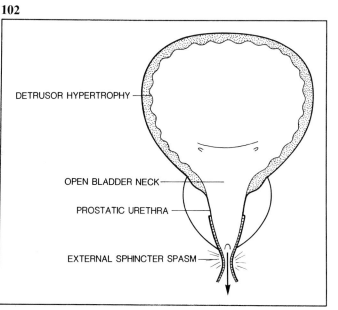

102 Spastic external sphincter.

103a Diagrammatic representation of normal male urethral pressure profile.

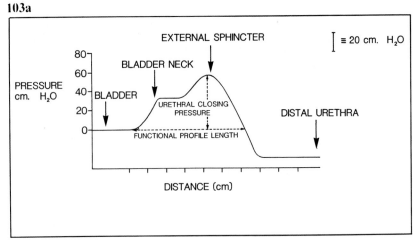

103b Urethral pressure profile – external sphincter spasm.

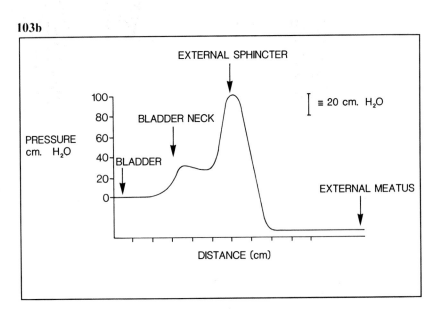

104 Urethral pressure profile – prostatic obstruction.

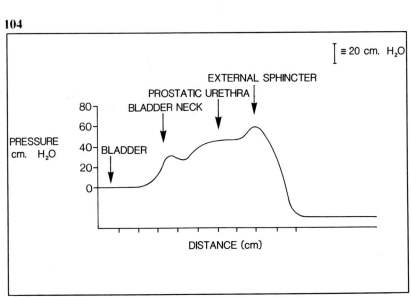

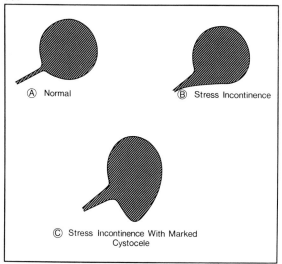

105

(A) Normal

(B) Stress Incontinence

(C) Stress Incontinence With Marked Cystocele

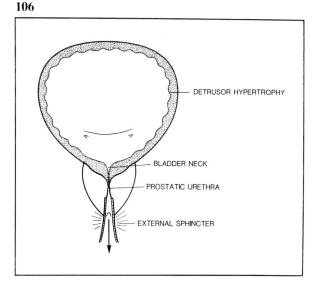

106

DETRUSOR HYPERTROPHY

BLADDER NECK

PROSTATIC URETHRA

EXTERNAL SPHINCTER

105　Cine appearances of lateral view of female bladder on coughing. Weakness of the pelvic floor in the female causes variable descent of the bladder base and proximal urethra; where support of the neck region is poor, stress incontinence results.

106　Prostatic obstruction.

Vesicoureteric reflux may be primary or secondary to outflow tract obstruction, with or without neurological bladder disease. Cine/pressure/flow studies aid full assessment and diagnosis.

107　Pressure-flow study of prostatic obstruction. This trace shows the high bladder pressure and poor flow rate in prostatic obstruction.

Outflow obstruction produced by bladder neck hypertrophy or prostatic intrusion into the urethra results in detrusor hypertrophy with high pressure contractions, low flow rate and poor opening of the neck or proximal urethra during micturition.

107

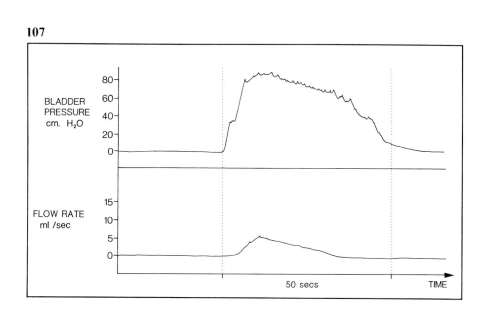

BLADDER PRESSURE cm. H_2O

80
60
40
20
0

FLOW RATE ml /sec

15
10
5
0

50 secs

TIME

2 Congenital abnormalities

Congenital abnormalities of the urinary tract are constantly seen and the variations are not only important but of great academic interest. Modern investigative techniques ensure that the correct diagnosis is made and enable the urologist to solve any problems that might otherwise escape his judgement. The importance of precise diagnosis cannot be stressed too strongly, because many congenital deformities of the renal tract predispose to disease to a far greater extent than those organs which have developed normally. Congenital deformities are more important for the complications they produce, rather than the inherent abnormality itself. Great care should be taken in their investigation, because multiple deformities in the urinary tract are not uncommon.

Presenting symptoms

Most congenital deformities are found on routine examination of vague symptoms related to the urinary tract. They may complain of loin or suprapubic pain, recurrent urinary tract infection or very occasionally painless haematuria. The first group of congenital abnormalities are presented according to the disturbances of embryological developments of the nephric system.

108 Diagram of the developing urinary system up to the fourth week (adapted from numerous sources).

At the fourth week the pronephros has almost completely disappeared, while mesonephric tubules have begun to form in the mesonephric duct. At this stage the earliest signs of the ureteric

bud arising from the mesonephric tissue can be seen.

The first group of conditions are caused by some failure in the normal development of the ureteric bud.

108

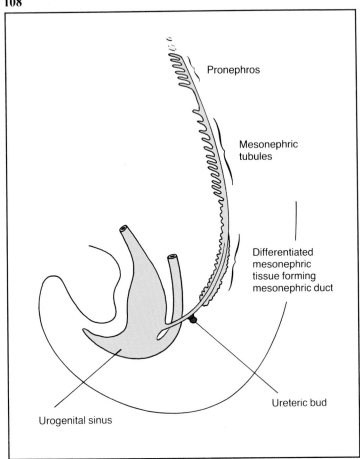

Pronephros

Mesonephric tubules

Differentiated mesonephric tissue forming mesonephric duct

Ureteric bud

Urogenital sinus

109

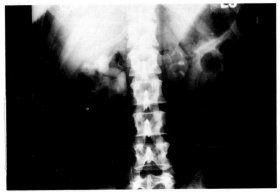

110

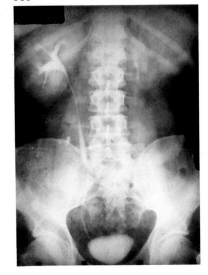

109 and 110 IVU of two hypoplastic kidneys which are small, shrunken and have very little cortex. This condition was probably caused by primary failure of the ureteric bud.

111

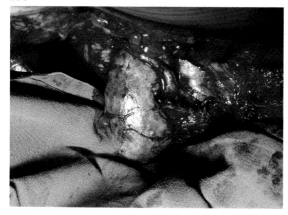

112

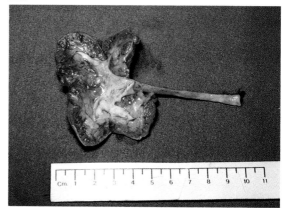

113

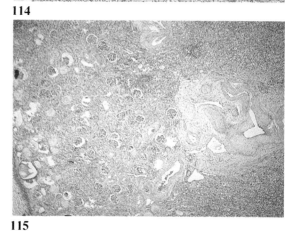

114

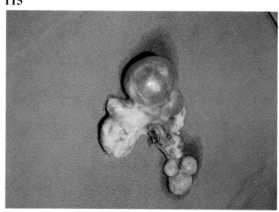

111 Hypoplastic kidney before nephrectomy. The kidney is small and of normal colour and shape.

112 Hypoplastic kidney. Section of same kidney showing thin cortex and very little functioning renal tissue. This kidney was discovered on routine examination for essential hypertension.

113 and 114 Hypoplastic kidney. Histology of same kidney. The sections show atrophy of the tubules, a heavy chronic inflammatory cell infiltrate in the interstitium and hypertensive changes in the vessels. These changes, together with the dilatation of some tubules and focal calcification, may be secondary.

115

115 Dysplastic kidney. This kidney is an example of the group of disorders in which abnormal metanephric differentiation is seen, frequently associated with cyst formation. The abnormal structures are recognised histologically (see **116** and **117**). Most cases described as aplastic, hypoplastic or multicystic kidney are really variants of this disorder.

116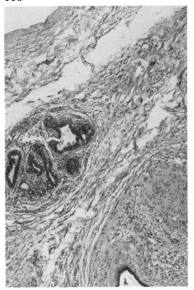

117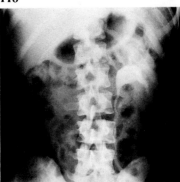

116 and 117 Dysplastic kidney. The pictures show an abnormal renal parenchyma with a paucity of nephrons. The abnormal ducts and tubules, lined by cuboidal to columnar epithelium which is sometimes ciliated are surrounded by cellular mesenchyme. Cartilage is sometimes present. The cysts are lined by flat epithelium.

Absent kidney

118 IVU showing no function of the right kidney.

119 Blind-ended ureter of absent kidney shown by ascending ureterogram. Most probably caused by the failure of the ureteric bud to make contact with the nephrogenic mesoderm.

118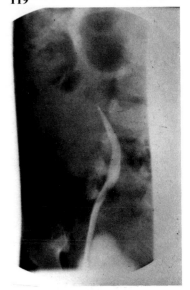

119

Absent kidney

Function

If the IVU shows no renal function a renal scan will confirm an absent kidney.

120 Scan on which no right kidney outline is seen.

Ectopic kidney

121

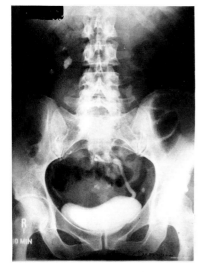

121a

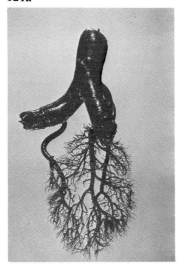

122

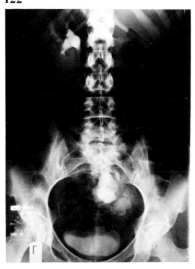

Ectopic kidney may be single or double, which it is suggested is caused by some coincidental vascular abnormality. They can be crossed with or without fusion which is due to the abnormal ascent of the ureteric bud.

121 Unilateral pelvic ectopic kidney with single ureter entering the bladder in the normal way.

121a Blood supply of ectopic kidney lying in the hollow of the skeletal pelvis. It is supplied by three arteries,

which bear no relationship to the pattern found in either normal or congenitally abnormal kidneys in the lumbar region. In this cast, the kidney was supplied by three arteries, two of which shared a common origin from the bifurcation of the aorta, while the third arose from the left common iliac artery. However, the blood supply of any pelvic ectopic kidney is very small.

122 Unilateral ectopic pelvic kidney with hydronephrosis caused by pelviureteric obstruction.

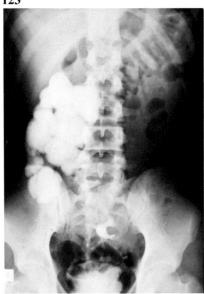

123 Unilateral ectopic left pelvic kidney with hydronephrosis of the right caused by pelviureteric obstruction.

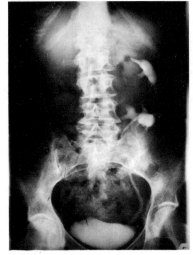

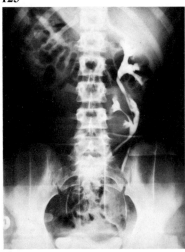

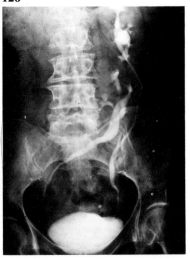

124 Crossed ectopic of one kidney fused with the kidney in the normal position which is rotated, but there are separate pelvicalyceal systems.

125 Crossed ectopic of one kidney fused with the other kidney with only one pelvicalyceal system.

126 Two separate crossed ectopic kidneys with separate pelvicalyceal systems.

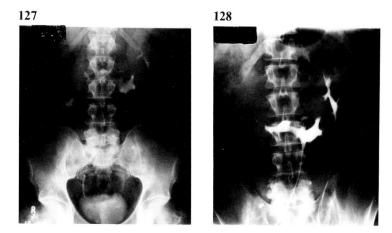

127 Two fused kidneys: right horseshoe, left rotated.

128 Retrograde pyelogram of the same patient.

128a

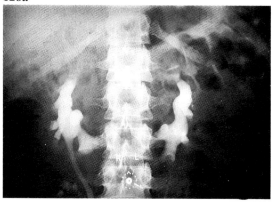

128a **Classical horseshoe kidney** for comparison (see page 48).

129

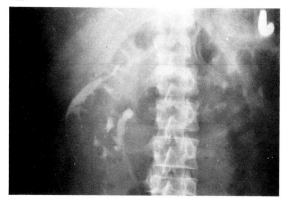

129 **Crossed ectopic with two fused kidneys** and one ureter opening into the urethra.

130 Embryological diagram of embryo at four weeks showing two ureteric buds. Ureteric anomalies account for about 30 per cent of all congenital abnormalities in the urinary tract; up to 10 per cent of all patients seen at urological clinics have some ureteric abnormality. The duplication of the ureter is caused by either early branching of the ascending ureter and its extent depends on the time when the ureter branches or the second ureteric bud which arises from the mesonephric duct. This diagram, which is only a very little older than the first, shows two ureteric buds and this is the cause of a duplication in the urinary tract.

130

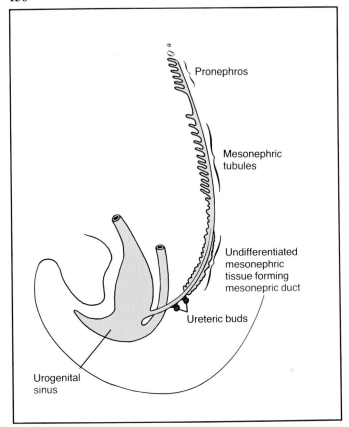

Pronephros

Mesonephric tubules

Undifferentiated mesonephric tissue forming mesonepric duct

Ureteric buds

Urogenital sinus

131

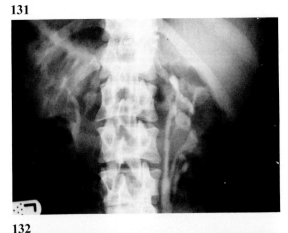

131 Bifid kidney. The division is in the upper third of the ureter and is caused by late branching of the ureteric ampulla. It is this condition which can give rise to abnormal peristalsis in the ureter leading to the 'yo-yo' flow of urine from one moiety to the other.

132

132 Duplex system starting at the upper third of the ureter indicative of late branching (arrowed).

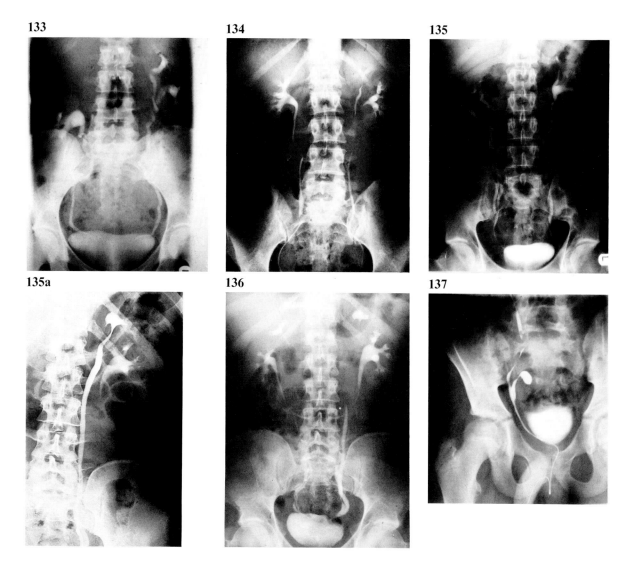

133   **Upper third duplex system** with the drooping lily appearance of the opposite side.

134   **Duplex system in which the two systems join in the middle third** of the ureter indicating earlier branching of the ureteric bud.

135 and 135a   **Mid-third ureteric duplication** with a small upper kidney moiety as a result of most branches of the ureteric bud joining with one moiety.

136   **Lower-third ureteric duplication** with one small kidney moiety.

137   **Retrograde pyelogram of lower-third ureteric duplication** in which one ureter opens into an ectopic hypoplastic kidney as a result of failure of development of one of the duplicated ureters.

138 Complete duplex system in which the ureters open separately into the bladder. Note the larger kidneys which are common in this condition, and there is also a higher incidence of multiple renal vessels.

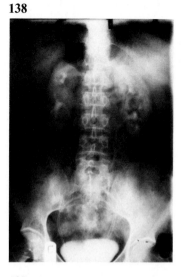

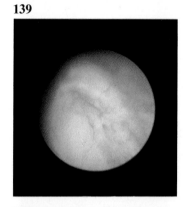

139 Duplex ureteric orifices. The upper orifice is always from the lower moiety. The hooded type of orifice is the one most likely to reflux.

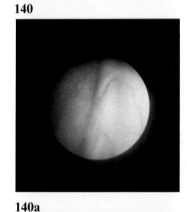

140 and 140a Further views of duplex ureteric orifices.

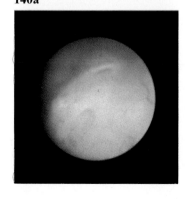

141

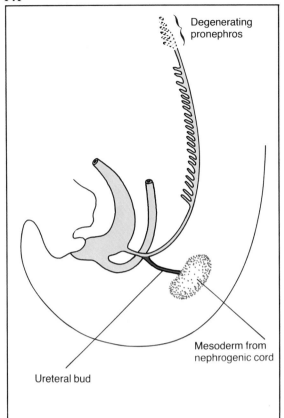

Degenerating
pronephros

Mesoderm from
nephrogenic cord

Ureteral bud

142

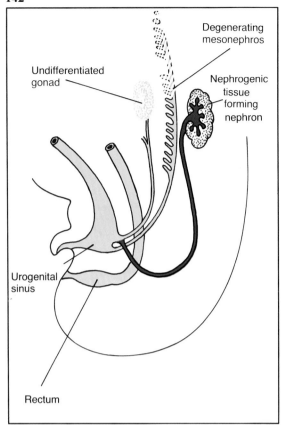

Degenerating
mesonephros

Undifferentiated
gonad

Nephrogenic
tissue
forming
nephron

Urogenital
sinus

Rectum

141   Embryological diagram of embryo at sixth week.
The pronephros is degenerating and the ureteric bud has
now joined the mesoderm from the nephrogenic cord;
the mesonephric duct moves caudally to be absorbed
into the vesicourethral area.

142   Embryological diagram of embryo at eight weeks.
At this time the cloaca has differentiated into the urinary
and lower bowel systems. The ureter, with its cap of
mesoderm, has moved caudally and the undifferentiated
gonads are first seen.

Malrotation is not an uncommon finding. The calyces
usually point vertically rather than laterally. The
condition rarely causes any problems.

143

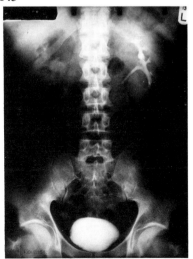

143   Ventral rotation of the renal pelvis caused by
failure of rotation during renal ascent.

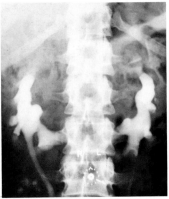
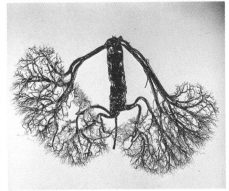
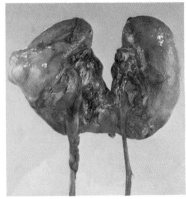

Abnormalities of fusion

Fusion is usually in the lower poles. The cause of this is probably an abnormality in ascent combined with some vascular abnormality, which leads to the lower poles failing to migrate laterally.

144a The horseshoe kidney which is the commonest variety of renal fusion. The union is at the lower pole and a bridge of renal tissue crosses in front of the aorta, spine and inferior vena cava. The long axes are parallel to the spine and there is an associated malrotation, the renal pelves lying anterior with the calyces posteriorly, laterally or medially.

A characteristic feature which is pathognomonic of a horseshoe kidney is the medially directed lower calyces passing to the bridge of renal tissue. The unusual relation of the renal vessels sometimes leads to obstruction which results in infection, hydronephrosis, occasionally stone formation or a combination of all three.

144b Blood supply – horseshoe kidney. The arteries to the apical, upper middle and posterior segments on either side of the aorta are of the same pattern as those of normal kidneys. The right lower segmental arteries, however, have not only arisen from a common trunk, but the posterior branches of these vessels have arisen earlier than the anterior branches and almost directly from the aorta.

144c Horseshoe kidney. The specimen shows the lower poles fused across the mid-line and the ureters passing down anteriorly.

145 Horseshoe kidney with hydronephrosis of one kidney caused by ureteric obstruction usually at the pelviureteric junction.

146 Horseshoe kidney in the lower pole of a bilateral duplex system, the upper moiety on the left side having been removed.

Complications of horseshoe kidneys

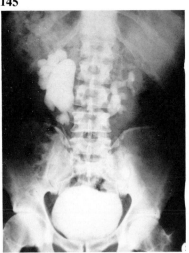
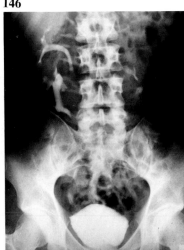
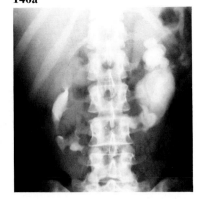

146a Small stones are not uncommon, but staghorn calculi producing obstruction as shown here are rare.

Complications of horseshoe kidney

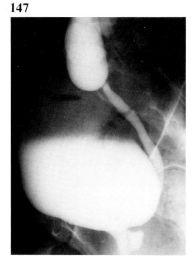

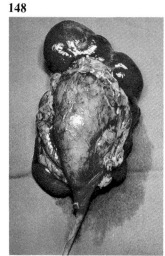

147 Ureteric reflux. Same patient with ureteric reflux into the left half of a horseshoe kidney.

148 Resected specimen showing dilated pelvis and diminished renal parenchyma, caused by persistent reflux and chronic recurrent infection.

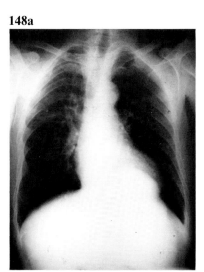

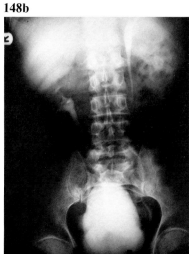

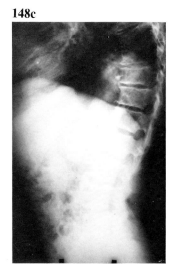

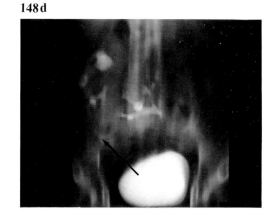

148a, b and c A thoracic kidney showing an abnormality of ascent. **148a** shows the diaphragmatic defect and the thoracic kidney is shown in the antero-posterior and lateral views.

148d An L-shaped kidney with a calculus in the right ureter.

148e and f A very unusual abnormality of formation of the pelvicalyceal system showing a blind calyx coming off from the front of the pelvis. Ultrasound arteriogram failed to show any renal substance attached to this single calyceal stem, so one must assume that it is a blind calyceal bud which has failed to join up with any renal parenchyma.

148e

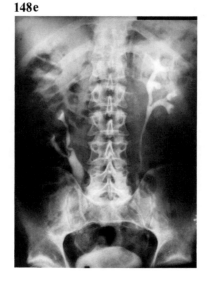

148f

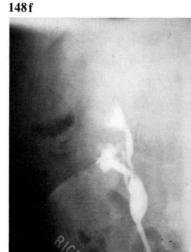

Other congenital abnormalities: cystic changes

149 Simple calyceal cyst which is probably caused by the defective final branching of the ureteric bud.

149

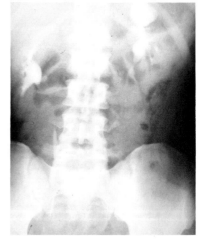

Multicystic disease

Multicystic disease is a rare condition manifested by multiple cysts often calcified.

150 IVU showing multiple cysts with peripheral calcification.

151 Arteriogram of the same patient showing avascular areas.

150

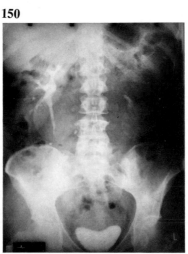

151

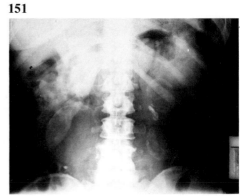

50

152

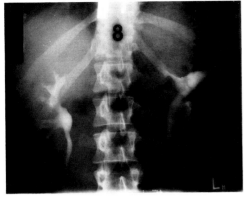

153

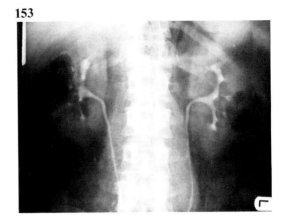

Polycystic disease (see Chapter 7 page 174)

Polycystic disease occurs in two major forms. Both have a hereditary basis and both involve all parts of both kidneys. The adult type (autosomal dominant, though many are new mutations), usually presents in adult life with hypertension and renal failure or haematuria. The kidneys are often massively enlarged. The infantile form (autosomal recessive) gives kidneys which cannot support life; death occurs early.

152 An example of polycystic disease showing the stretched pelvicalyceal system, the enlarged kidneys with irregular surface and the deformity of the calyces caused by the pressure of the cysts.

153 Further example of polycystic disease.

154

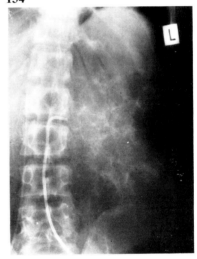

154 and 155 Two different phases of an arteriogram of a polycystic kidney in which the vascular pattern is completely distorted.

155

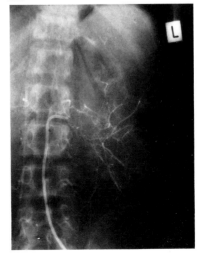

156

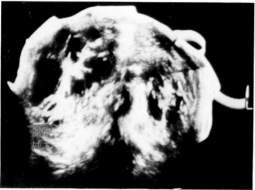

157

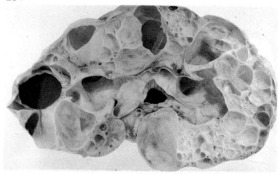

157a

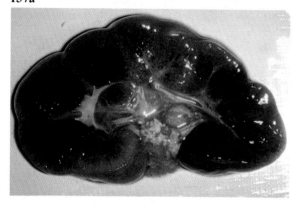

158

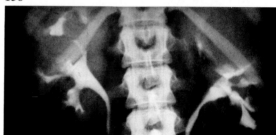

159

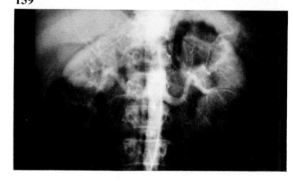

156 Ultrasound of polycystic kidney in which the cystic areas are clearly shown.

157 Adult type polycystic kidney. This is a formalin-fixed specimen from a postmortem of a young adult dying of a cerebral haemorrhage associated with hypertension. Both kidneys were like this one. (They are very much larger than the infantile polycystic.)

157a Infantile polycystic kidneys. This form of polycystic disease results in kidneys that cannot support life. Cystically dilated tubules radiate from the pelvis to the cortex. The specimen was taken from an infant that died within two days of birth.

158 IVU of a polycystic kidney in which a carcinoma has developed on the lower pole distorting the calyces and the pelvis.

159 Arteriogram showing the avascular upper pole caused by the cyst and the tumour blush in the tumour.

160 Arteriogram/nephrogram phase confirming lower pole tumour.

160a Medullary sponge kidney. The specimen shows multiple small cysts in the medulla. There is a little scarring of the cortex, possibly caused by secondary infection. It was an incidental finding at postmortem of an elderly lady who died from an unrelated disease.

160a

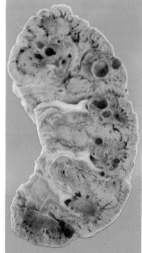

160

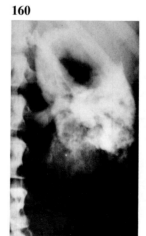

161

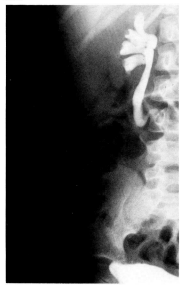

162

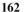
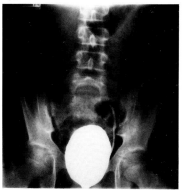

163

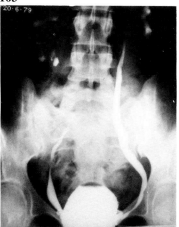

164

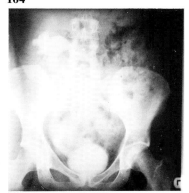

Retrocaval ureter

Retrocaval ureter is caused by persistence of the precursor of the inferior vena cava remaining anterior to the ureter.

161 **Retrocaval ureter** in which the characteristic curve of the ureter is clearly seen.

Ureteric reflux (see Chapter 3 pages 69 and 70)

Ureteric reflux is divided into three categories – 1 Affecting only the lower third of the ureter; 2 Affecting up to the pelvicalyceal system; 3 When the reflux fills and dilates the ureter and pelvicalyceal system. It is diagnosed by a micturating cystogram, films being taken during straining and during and after micturition.

162 **Grade I reflux.**

163 **Grade II reflux.**

164 **Grade III reflux.**

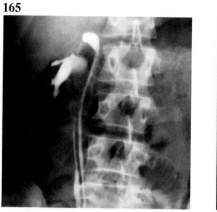

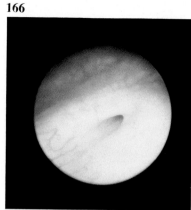

165 **Grade III reflux** into a complete duplex system with atrophy of the upper moiety.

166 **Refluxing ureteric orifice** which is gaping, hooded and pale. The contraction of this type of orifice is usually weak.

Ureterocele

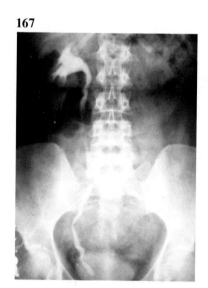

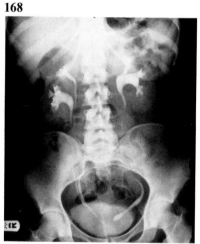

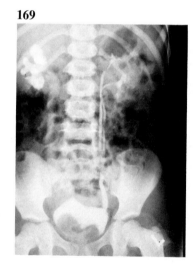

A ureterocele is a congenital cystic dilatation of the submucosal segment of the lower end of the ureter. It can be unilateral or bilateral, simple or part of a duplex system, or ectopic. The basic embryological disturbance is probably some malformation when the ureteric bud is forming the ureteric orifice in the degenerating mesonephric duct.

167 **Unilateral ureterocele** showing classical cobra-head appearance.

168 **Bilateral ureterocele**, the right being from the upper moiety of a duplex system.

169 **Unilateral ureterocele** affecting upper moiety of the duplex system with reflux into the lower moiety.

169a

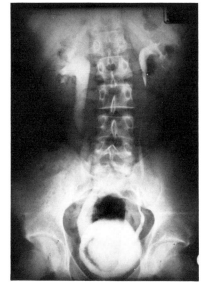

170

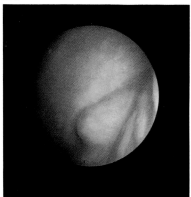

170 Ureterocele showing dilated thin mucosa.

169a Ureteroceles can vary in size even in the same patient. IVU shows large right ureterocele and small classical left cobra-head ureterocele.

170a

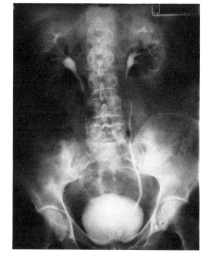

170b

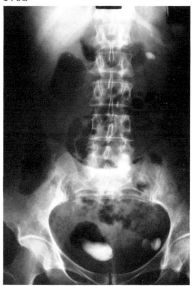

170c

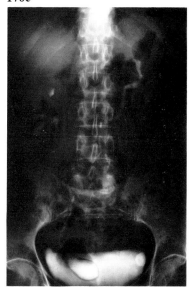

170a Small ureterocele with a calculus in situ.

170b and c KUB and IVU: Stones can become quite large.

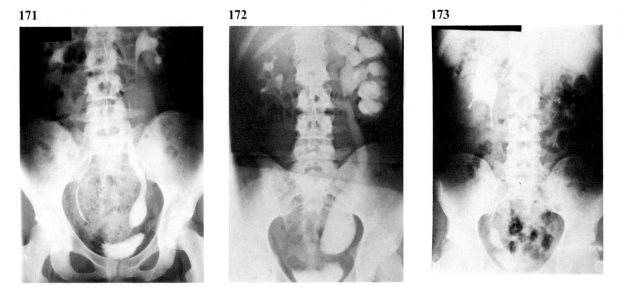

171   **172**   **173**

Functional obstruction

Obstruction at the lower end of the ureter which caused dilatation of the ureter ending in a thin taper, yet on intravenous urography allows a ureteric catheter to pass up unhindered is not uncommon and may be associated with and obstruction at the pelviureteric junction. It may be bilateral or unilateral.

171   **Early functional lower ureteric obstruction.** This obstruction may remain unchanged and symptomless for many years.

172   **A more pronounced obstruction** producing back pressure in the kidney causing dilatation of the pelvicalyceal system.

173   **Lower ureteric obstruction** combined with early pelviureteric obstruction.

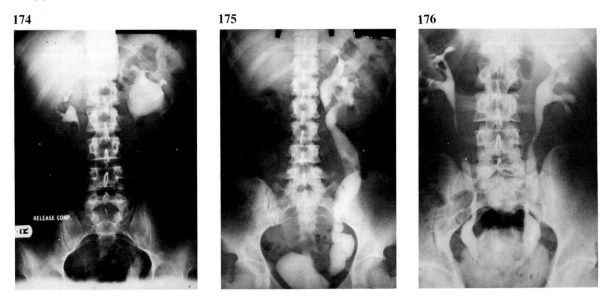

174   **175**   **176**

174   **Lower ureteric obstruction** combined with well marked pelviureteric obstruction.

175   **Functional lower ureteric obstruction:** the late effects.

176   **Bilateral functioning lower ureteric obstruction** with normal upper urinary tract.

177a

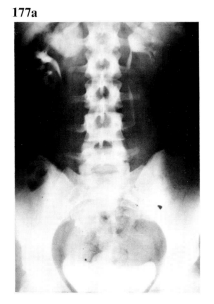

177b

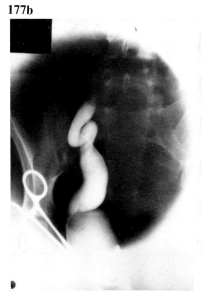

177a and b A large dilated upper moiety of a duplex kidney. Showing a large hydronephrosis of this moiety and the dilated lower ureter.

Pelviureteric obstruction

Pelviureteric obstruction may present in many ways and may be unilateral or bilateral.

Investigations

1 Renal scanning and renography. These investigations should be considered as complementary to intravenous urography, but they are non-invasive techniques and can give valuable information.

178, 179 and 180 Scintogram of hypotonic renal pelvis, 5, 25 and 30 minutes after injection of 1^{123} sodium iodohippurate, showing retention of the isotope in the pelvis and calyces of the left kidney.

178

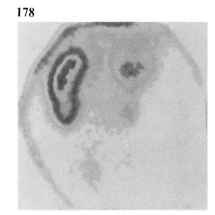

179

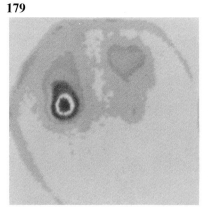

180

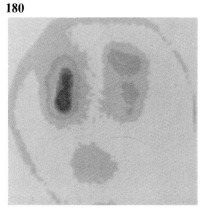

Renography

Renography is a means of monitoring the arrival uptake and removal of the radioisotope from the kidneys to give a reasonable assessment of the function of each kidney.

181 Renogram showing a normal right kidney pattern but the pattern of an obstructed left kidney. It is important to know whether hydronephrosis is caused by a hypotonic pelvis or a pelviureteric obstruction. In most cases a frusemide diuretic renogram will differentiate between the two conditions.

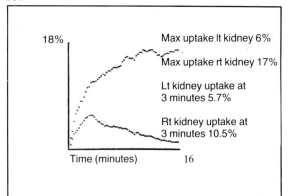

182 Diuretic renogram showing an obstructive lesion which does not resolve after frusemide administration indicating that surgery may be required.

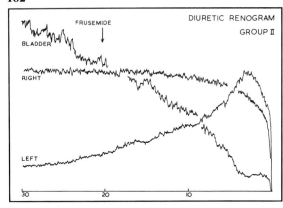

183 Diuretic renogram which demonstrates the rapid elimination of the radionuclide, often indicating that there is no pelviureteric obstruction.

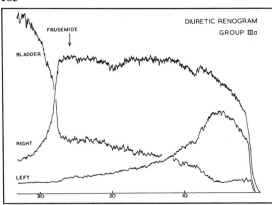

184 The diuresis renogram in this patient is equivocal, suggesting a combination of hypotonicity and some pelviureteric obstruction.

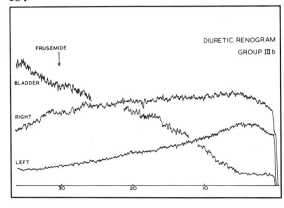

The Whitaker test

The Whitaker test can also be used for differentiating between an obstruction at the pelviureteric junction and a hypotonic pelvis.

185 and 186 are two cases of hydronephrosis. **185** is obstructed as **187** shows an obstructed tracing on the Whitaker test and so requires surgery, while **188** shows an unobstructed tracing.

185

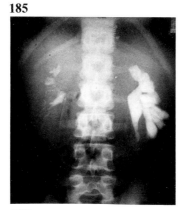

186

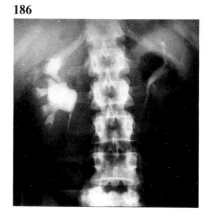

187

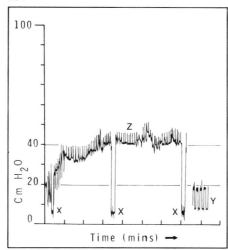

188

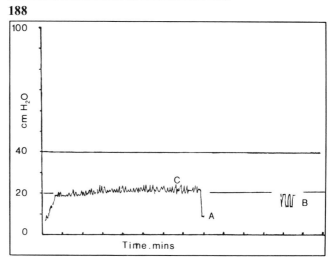

Ultrasound

Ultrasound has very little place in the initial investigations of a case of suspected hydronephrosis, but it may be of value for assessing progress at the time of follow-up examination.

189a and b: 190a and b Transverse and lateral ultrasound of a case of bilateral hydronephrosis demonstrating hydrocalycosis, the right kidney being worse than the left.

189a

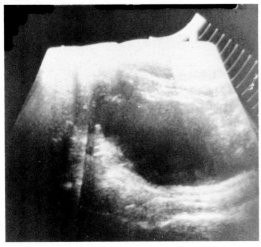

189b

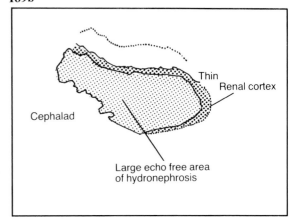

190a

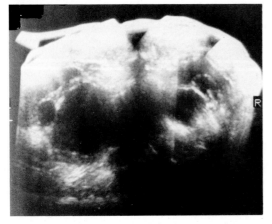

190b

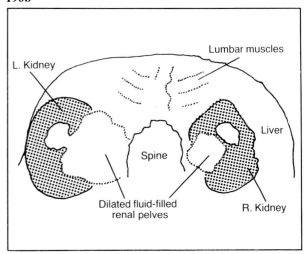

Urography

Intravenous urography is the most important investigation, but occasionally a retrograde pyelogram is required when there is a hydronephrotic kidney on one side and a non-functioning kidney on the other.

191 Intravenous urogram of a hydronephrotic right kidney with no function on the left.

192 Tomogram which reveals a large left renal outline.

193 and 194 Bilateral retrograde pyelogram confirming bilateral hydronephrosis.

195 Pelviureteric junction obstruction, due to vessel crossing the ureter causing the pelvis to fall over the ureter which then becomes acutely kinked, resulting in progressive hydronephrosis.

191

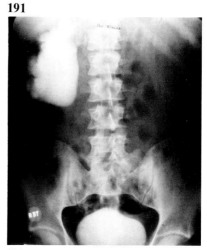

192

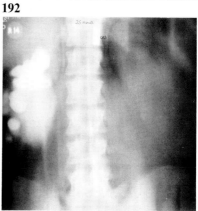

193

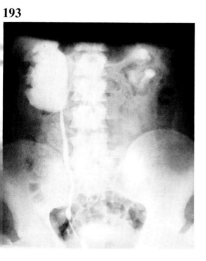

194

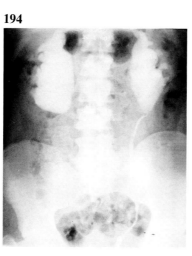

195

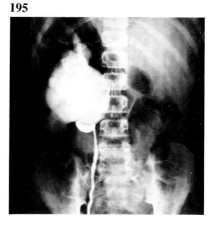

196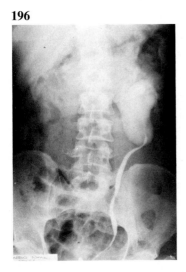

197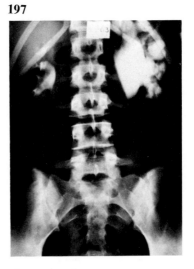

198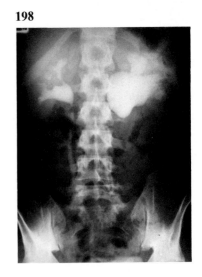

196 Pelviureteric junction obstruction showing elongated type of pelvis. With high take off of ureter from pelvis.

197 Hydronephrosis causing marked dilatation of the calyces with minimal distension of the pelvis.

198 Hydronephrosis with distorted calyces and funnel-shaped pelvis.

199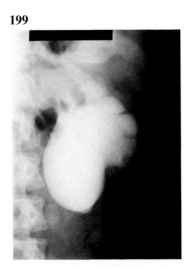

200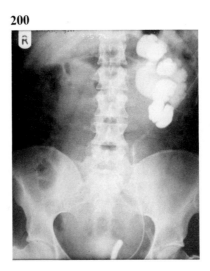

201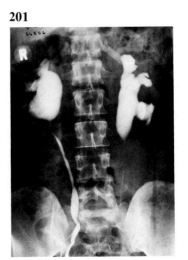

199 Considerable pelvic hydronephrosis with very early calyceal dilatation.

200 Considerable pelvic hydronephrosis with more advanced calyceal dilatation.

201 Bilateral pelviureteric obstruction.

202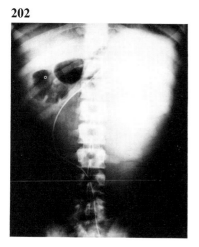

203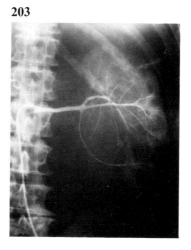

204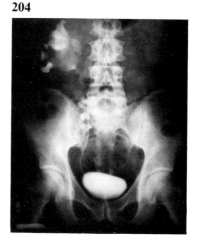

The hydronephrosis may become extremely large

202 Gross hydronephrosis pushing the ureter across the midline.

203 Selective renal arteriogram showing a large dilated pelvis distorting the arterial system. The lower branch of the renal artery is coursing round the large hydronephrotic pelvis.

Complications of pelviureteric obstruction

Infection is one the complications of pelviureteric obstruction.

204 Pelviureteric obstruction with a filling defect in the pelvis caused by mucopus. Obstruction can eventually lead to total destruction of the kidney.

205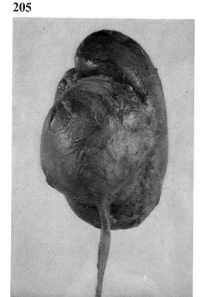

205a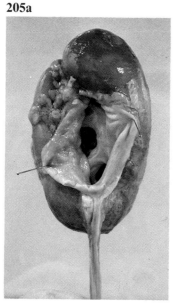

206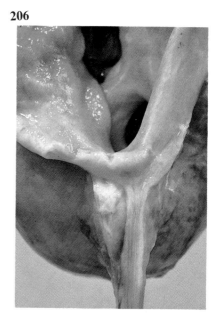

205, 205a and 206 Pelviureteric obstruction. Three pictures of the same hydronephrotic kidney. **205** shows the unopened specimen showing the dilatation above the pelviureteric junction (PUJ). **205a** demonstrates the opened pelvis and ureter with no anatomical structural lesion at the PUJ. **206** is a close-up of the PUJ with the dilated pelvicalyceal system above.

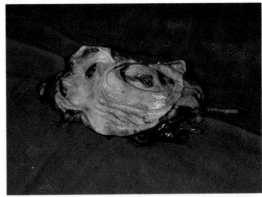

207 and 208 Typical longstanding obstruction which has destroyed the renal parenchyma, so that only a thin shell of renal tissue remains. Repeated attacks of infection lead to pyonephrosis which will rapidly destroy the kidney.

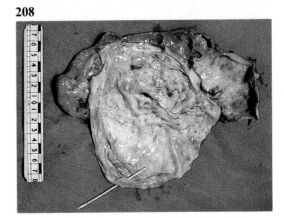

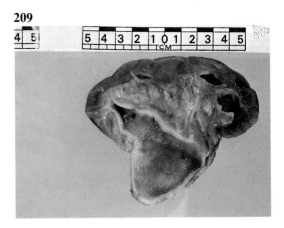

209 A kidney completely destroyed by repeated attacks of infection.

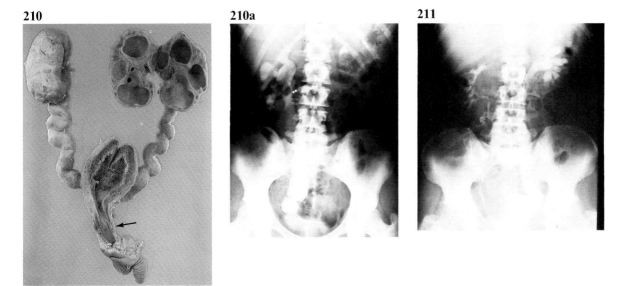

210 Urethral valve. A specimen from a male infant who died 10 days after birth. There are two folds extending laterally from the urethral crest, forming cusps just above the membranous urethra. These have acted as valves resulting in hypertrophy of the urethra and bladder above them. Hydroureter and hydronephrosis are present, with atrophy of the renal parenchyma.

Congenital megaureter

210a Congenital megaureter with minimal renal damage.

211 Congenital megaureter with commencing renal damage.

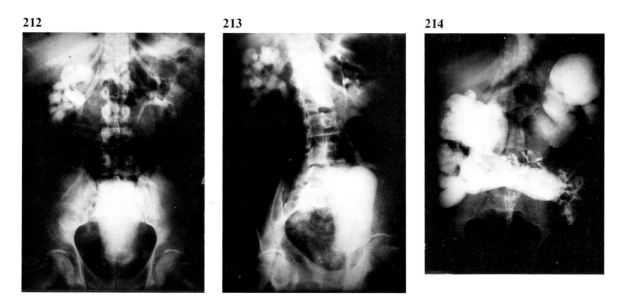

Pelvic lipomatosis

This is a condition of unknown origin in which the pelvis is filled by lipomatous tissue.

212 Bladder elevated, right ureter obstructed causing early hydronephrosis. Note the dark shadow in the pelvis.

213 Oblique view of the same patient.

214 Barium enema to show the rectal string sign caused by external pressure of the lipomatous tissue (dark shadow) on the rectum.

3 Inflammatory diseases of the urinary tract

Pyelonephritis

Acute bacterial pyelonephritis is usually a dramatic febrile illness, presenting with loin pain and rigors. Chronic bacterial pyelonephritis is insidious and may lead to hypertension and renal failure: it rarely occurs unless an abnormality exists somewhere in the outflow tract. Bacteria may reach the kidney by the bloodstream, lymph or via the ureter, but it is likely that most are ascending infections. The bacteria involved are usually gram-negative bacilli, particularly Escherichia coli (E. coli) and Bacillus proteus, but may also be caused by gram-positive organisms including Streptococcus faecalis and Staphylococcus albus. These organisms can produce inflammatory disorders at all levels of the urinary tract.

'Chronic pyelonephritis' has been an over diagnosed condition because of the assumption that all coarsely scarred kidneys result from urinary tract infection. This is not so; similar changes can result from vascular abnormalities, analgesic abuse or irradiation. In the absence of obstruction or proof of infection, it is better to use the term 'interstitial nephritis' for such kidneys.

This section also includes parasitic infestations such as bilharzia, chyluria and the inflammatory conditions produced by specific disease such as diabetes and analgesic abuse. The rarer conditions of obscure aetiology such as interstitial cystitis, retroperitoneal fibrosis and malakoplakia are also presented.

215

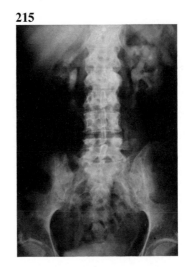

216

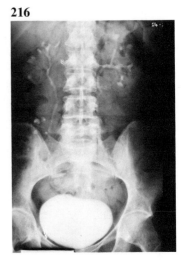

215 IVU showing severe bilateral pyelonephritis with reduction in kidney size, cortical scarring and calyceal dilatation and deformity.

216 IVU showing less marked bilateral changes.

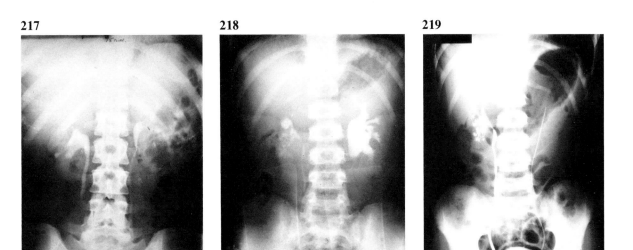

217   Changes may be much less severe and a scar with a related superficial calyx in the right kidney indicates focal damage.

218 and 219   When there is only minimal function in the IVU, here on the right side, retrograde pyelography will delineate the small, severely damaged kidney.

220   Changes may be confined to one pole and often seen affecting the upper pole as in this IVU.

220

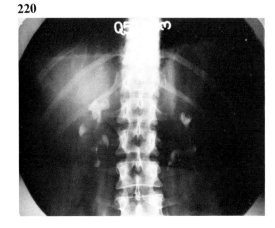

221 **222** **223**

221 **Calyceal clubbing** is well demonstrated here (see 227).

222 **Calyceal clubbing.** The severity of the process often varies between the two kidneys.

223 **Calyceal clubbing.** Sometimes the disease process may be effectively unilateral.

224

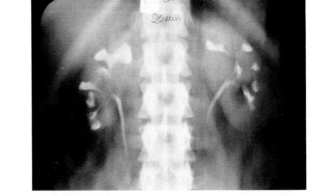

224 **Pyelonephritis** in children and adolescent females gives rise to the suspicion of primary vesicoureteric reflux. This IVU shows classical cortical thinning and calyceal damage in a 19-year-old girl with a history of 10 years' urinary tract infections.

Micturating cystourethrogram
(MCU)

225

226

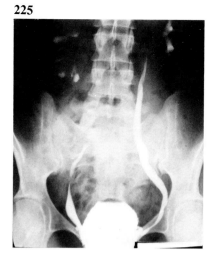
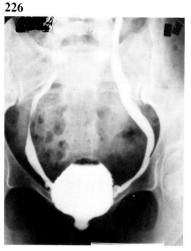

225 and 226   The micturating cystogram is an essential investigation in all such patients with recurrent urinary tract infection. Reflux is recorded in three grades (see **227**). Here early Grade III bilateral reflux is shown.

227   Three grades of reflux. Grade I in which contrast medium enters the ureter only. Grade II in which the pelvicalyceal system is filled with dye. Grade III where dilatation of calyces and ureter also occurs in varying degrees. This shows gross calyceal clubbing.

227

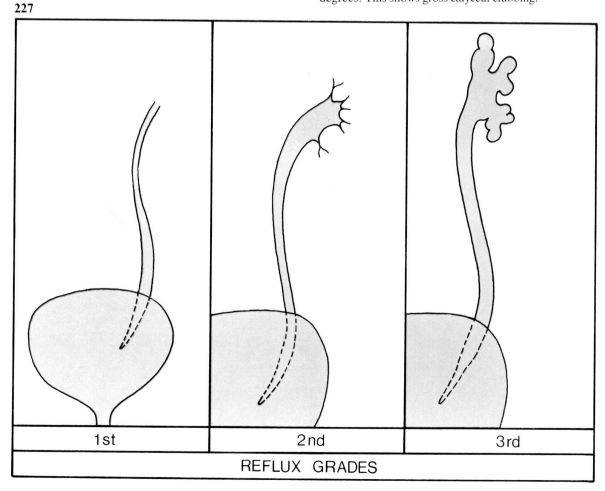

1st	2nd	3rd
REFLUX GRADES		

228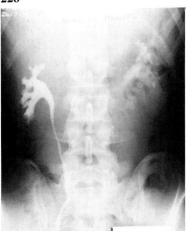

229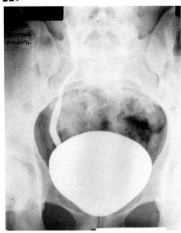

230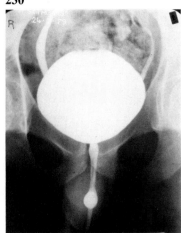

228 **Bilateral reflux** may not cause severe renal changes as in this MCU of a young male.

229 **Low pressure reflux.** During the filling phase of the MCU Grade I low pressure reflux is seen on the right.

230 **High pressure reflux.** On voiding, bilateral high pressure reflux occurs.

231 **Grade III reflux is demonstrated.**

232 **IVU showing right duplex system** with ureterocele and normal left system.

232a **Congenital anatomical ureteric anomalies** may also give rise to reflux. This young woman had a complete right duplex ureteric system. Reflux is seen into the lower moiety of the right kidney with that ureter entering the bladder above the upper moiety ureter. This second ureter terminated in a small ureterocele with obstruction. No reflux nor obstruction occurred on the left side.

231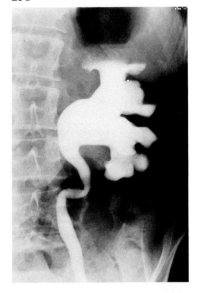

232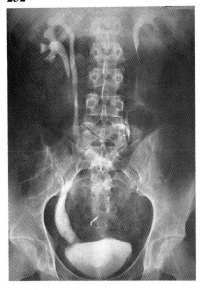

232a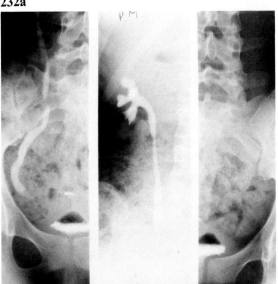

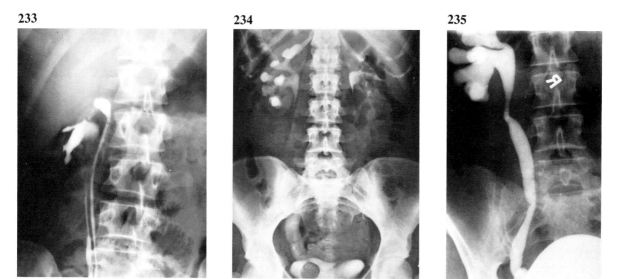

233 Reflux may also occur in both ureters of a duplex system.

234 and 235 Reflux may also be secondary to iatrogenic damage to the ureteric orifices in endoscopic procedures and here followed endoscopic incision of a ureterocele.

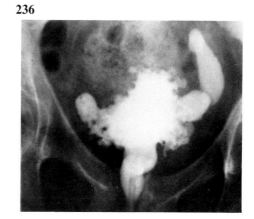

236 Also as a result of obstruction to the lower tract or in neuropathic bladder disorders, as seen here.

237

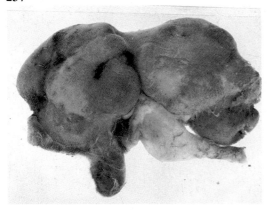

238

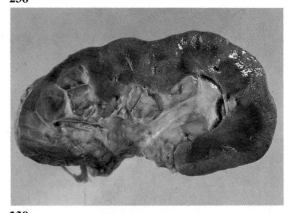

239

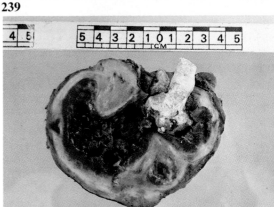

240

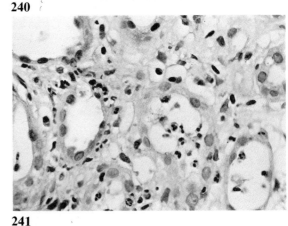

241

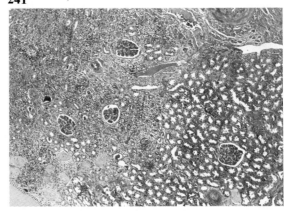

237 Chronic pyelonephritis. Outer surface of a coarsely scarred kidney (formalin fixed).

238 Chronic pyelonephritis. Cut surface of a coarsely scarred kidney showing distortion of the pelvicalyceal system and loss of renal parenchyma in the scarred areas.

239 Xanthogranulomatous pyelonephritis. This kidney contains a staghorn calculus. The pelvis is dilated and haemorrhagic. The renal parenchyma is scarred and contains yellow-orange areas. Histology of these areas shows many lipid-laden histiocytes with multinucleate giant cells, the pattern of xanthogranulomatous pyelonephritis. See also **250**.

240 Acute pyelonephritis. Section from a patient with proven urinary tract infection, showing neutrophil poly-morphonuclear leucocyte infiltration of the tubular epithelium and lumen. *(H&E × 256)*

241 Chronic pyelonephritis. Section showing an area of relatively normal parenchyma (on the righthand side of the field) with a very abnormal one (on the left). In the abnormal area the striking feature is the tubular damage and inflammatory cell infiltrate in the interstitium. Three relatively well-preserved glomeruli are present in the middle of this area, but some sclerotic ones are present in the bottom lefthand corner. This patchy involvement is a feature of chronic pyelonephritis. *(H&E × 26)*

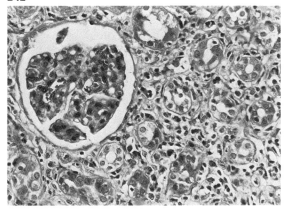

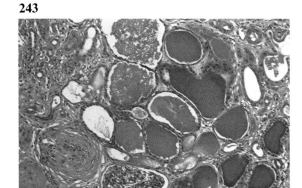

242 Chronic pyelonephritis. A higher magnification of **241** showing chronic inflammatory cell infiltration in the interstitium with a preserved glomerulus. *(H&E × 160)*

243 Chronic pyelonephritis. Marked tubular dilatation, the lumens being filled with eosinophilic protein casts. This appearance is similar to the colloid-filled follicles in the thyroid and is often called thyroidisation. *(H&E × 64)*

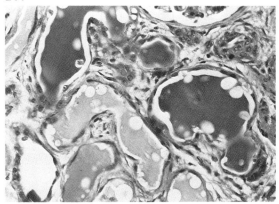

244 Chronic pyelonephritis. Higher magnification of tubules similar to those in **243**, showing the marked flattening of the tubular epithelium. *(H&E × 160)*

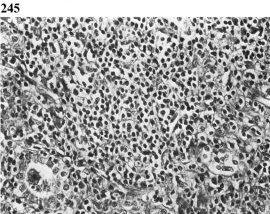

245 Chronic pyelonephritis. A section of medulla showing marked infiltration of the interstitium with inflammatory cells, with some entering the tubules. *(H&E × 160)*

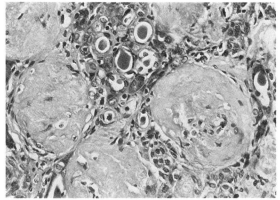

246 Chronic pyelonephritis. In an advanced stage scarring and hyalinisation may predominate over inflammatory cell infiltration. This section shows hyalinised glomeruli and some protein casts in atrophic tubules. *(H&E × 160)*

247 Chronic pyelonephritis. Arterial changes are often prominent, especially in advanced disease. This section shows an artery with marked intimal proliferation in the middle of the field. Some hyalinised glomeruli are present. In advanced disease it may be difficult to decide whether the process is infective in origin. *(H&E × 160)*

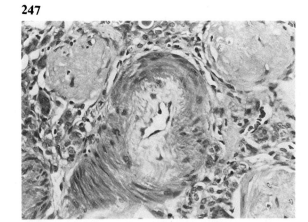

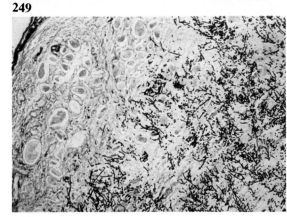

248 and 249 Fungal infections may also cause renal inflammatory disease as in candidiasis of the kidney. Renal candidiasis presenting as a Candida ball usually results from a widespread overwhelming fungal infection in the seriously debilitated patient. **248** shows budding forms of candida albicans. **249** is a silver preparation showing fungal hyphae (black) growing in tissue.

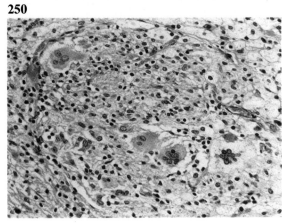

250 Xanthogranulomatous pyelonephritis is a term applied to a form of chronic pyelonephritis where a heavy infiltrate of histiocytes (macrophages) is prominent among the chronic inflammatory cells. These cells have foamy cytoplasm, caused by their lipid content, and some are multinucleate. The appearances are similar to those seen in a xanthoma, which usually lacks other inflammatory cells. *(H&E × 80)*

251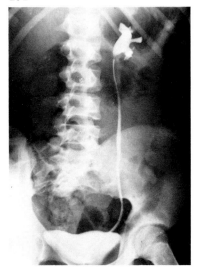

252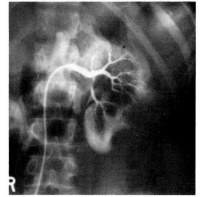

253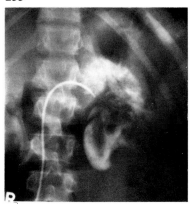

251 Abscess formation may occur in distinct areas of the renal cortex producing a renal carbuncle which is usually staphylococcal in origin, but may be secondary to suppurative pyelonephritis. Notoriously difficult to diagnose, the patients are ill, febrile, often develop flank pain late and the urine may be sterile. Pyelography and retrograde studies may be unhelpful although pelvicalyceal distortion may occur and the renal outline be altered.

252 and 253 Arteriography demonstrates here an irregular loss of renal tissue at the lower pole.

Perinephric abscess

Almost always arising from the kidney and most frequently in association with stone disease, the abscess lies around the kidney, usually confined by Gerota's fascia, and may point through the skin or drain into the colon. Occasionally it may track below the inguinal ligament or up to the diaphragm.

254

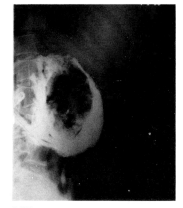

254 A gas filled abscess cavity is seen.

255

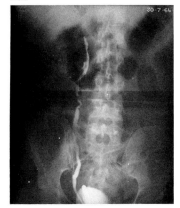

255 Retrograde study shows compression and medial deviation of the pelvicalyceal system.

256 Pyonephrotic kidney: outer surface. Pyonephrosis is normally a result of infection by pyogenic organisms after obstruction by stone or of a hydronephrotic kidney with pelviureteric obstruction. This leads to rapid destruction of the kidney.

256

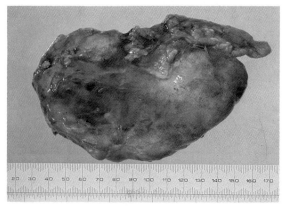

257

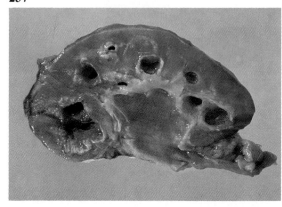

257 Pyonephrosis. The cut surface of the specimen shown in **256**. The dilated pelvis was filled with pus and abscesses are present in the renal parenchyma, communicating with the pelvis.

258

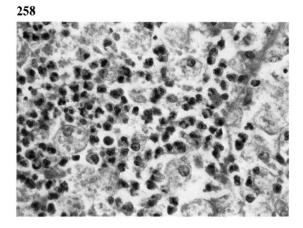

258 Pyonephrosis. Section from near the pelvis. It shows many neutrophil polymorphonuclear leucocytes with some larger cells with foamy cytoplasm (histiocytes with ingested material). *(H&E × 256)*

259

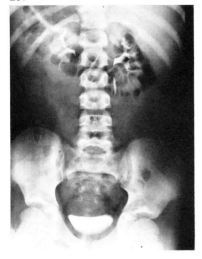

260

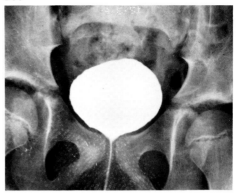

261

UTL F 8 yrs: Bladder infection	
Specimen	Bacterial count per ml
CU	Proteus mirabilis 10^6
WB	Proteus mirabilis 60 cols
RK1–5	No growth
LK1–5	No growth

259, 260 and 261 Localisation studies for bacterial infection are valuable for assessment of recurrent or chronic urinary tract infections. This child with recurrent urinary tract infection had a normal IVU, **259**, no reflux on the MCU, **260**, and localisation showed infection confined to the bladder alone, **261**.

262

UTL F 53 yrs: L renal infection, hypoplastic kidney	
Specimen	Bacterial count per ml
CU	Escherichia coli 10^6
WB	Escherichia coli 20 cols
RK1–5	No growth
LK1	Escherichia coli 10^4
LK2–5	Escherichia coli 10^6

263

UTL F 18 yrs: Bilateral renal infection	
Specimen	Bacterial count per ml
CU	Escherichia coli 10^8
WB	Escherichia coli 10^2
RK1–5	Escherichia coli 10^6
LK1–5	Escherichia coli 10^6

262 and 263 Upper tract infections may be unilateral or bilateral and are frequently associated with stone disease.

CU = Cystoscopic urine specimen.
WB = Washed bladder specimen.
RK/LK1–5 = 5 consecutive ureteric specimens of urine from each kidney.

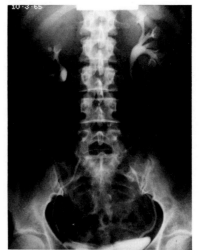

264

265

264, 265 and 266 **IVU essentially normal** but plain film shows small calculus in the left lower zone. Localisation study confirms left sided infection.

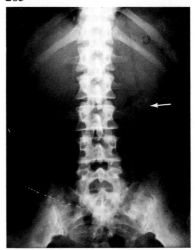

266

UTL F 42 yrs: L renal infection associated with stone

Specimen	Bacterial count per ml
CU	Proteus mirabilis 10^6
WB	No growth
RK1–5	No growth
LK1, 2	Proteus mirabilis 10^2
LK3	Proteus mirabilis 10^3
LK4, 5	Proteus mirabilis 10^{3-4}

267

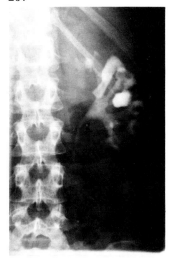

268

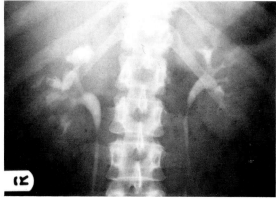

269

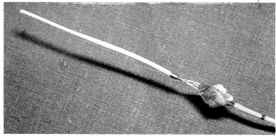

270

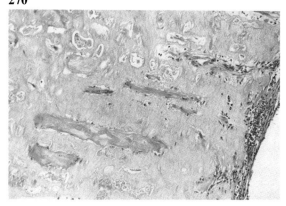

270a

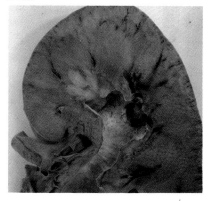

267 and 268 Papillary necrosis is most commonly associated with diabetes and analgesic abuse but may also occur in sickle cell disease. The IVU shows calyceal ulceration, scarring and clubbing. The classical ring negative shadow of the sloughed papilla is seen. **268** shows less marked changes.

269 The sloughed papilla causing ureteric obstruction, extracted endoscopically with the dormia basket.

270 Papillary necrosis. Section showing the structured necrosis seen in papillary necrosis. Note the ghost outlines of the structure of the papilla with virtual absence of nuclear staining. *(H&E × 26)*

270a Papillary necrosis. Postmortem specimen of a kidney from a diabetic patient. The extreme pallor of the papillae is caused by necrosis (formalin fixed).

271   **272**   **273**

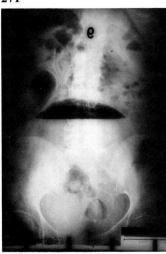 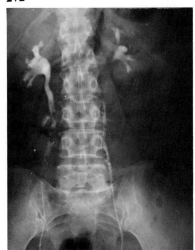 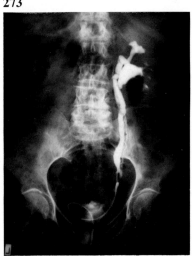

271   In diabetes, infection may occur with gas forming organisms giving rise to gas in the bladder, and here also in the right kidney.

272   Chronic bacterial infection may give rise to the pyelographic changes of pyelo-ureteritis cystica.

273   These may progress to marked ureteric changes with irregularity and filling defects, shown on the ascending study. The histological appearances are the same as those of cystitis cystica.

274

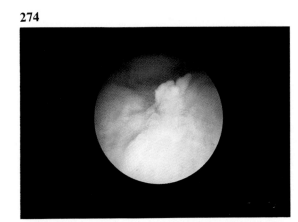

274   Intra-abdominal chronic inflammatory disease such as diverticulitis or Crohn's disease may lead to fistulation to the ureter or bladder. The characteristic granulations around the fistulous opening at endoscopy are seen.

275

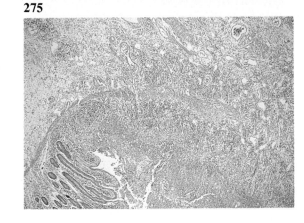

275   **Crohn's disease** is a chronic inflammatory disease of the alimentary tract, particularly affecting the terminal ileum. The cause is unknown, but the inflammation spreads right through the wall of the bowel and may penetrate into other organs including the bladder. This picture shows an ulcerated piece of small bowel mucosa with inflammation spreading into the wall. *(H&E)*

Idiopathic retroperitoneal fibrosis (RPF)

This condition, first described by Ormond in 1948, is a proliferation of fibrous tissue, often with blood vessels and other inflammatory cells. It develops in the retroperitoneum, usually centred around the aorta, often low down extending upwards and tends to involve the ureters, causing hydronephrosis and resulting in renal failure. Some similar cases are associated with methysergide therapy for migraine. It is important to remember that some neoplasms in the retroperitoneum can stimulate a fibroblastic response which can be mistaken for idiopathic RPF.

276 **277** **278**

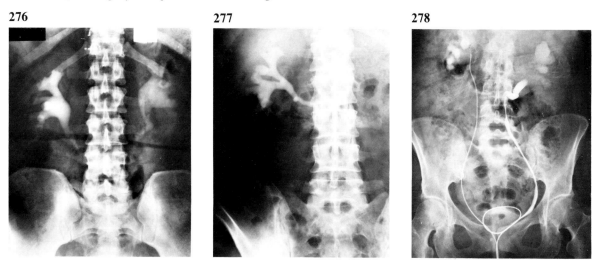

276 Bilateral hydronephrosis, typical of this condition, is seen in this IVU.

277 Gross medial indrawing of the ureter is present in this patient whose left kidney was removed earlier for 'hydronephrosis of unknown cause'.

278 Bilateral ureteric catheterisation shows the indrawn ureters, but catheters may pass without any difficulty.

279 **280** **281**

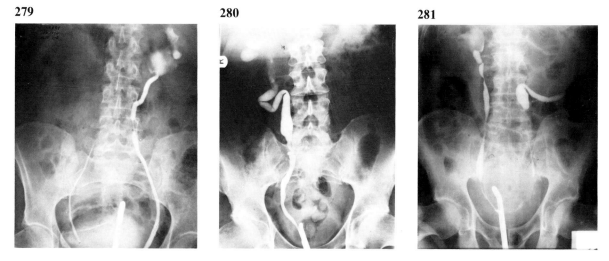

279 and 280 Ascending ureterography, using the bulb ended ureteric catheter, is diagnostic in that the extrinsic compression of the ureter by fibrosis is delineated.

281 A long ureteric stricture may also be found.

282 and 283 **Calcification** can occur in a plaque of retroperitoneal fibrosis, which may give rise to difficulty with diagnosis. Plain film and IVU.

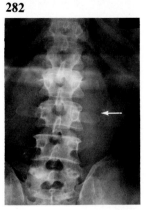

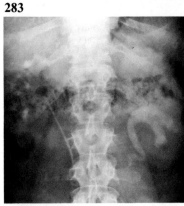

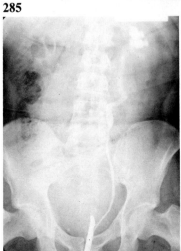

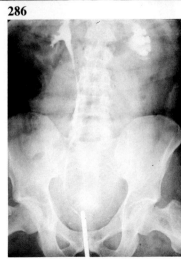

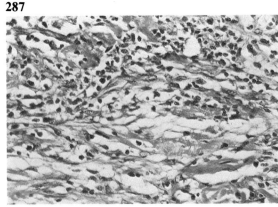

284, 285 and 286 Although the condition usually affects both ureters, it can present with unilateral obstruction. The IVU and left ascending ureterogram demonstrate RPF affecting the left ureter while the right ureterogram is normal. Exploration and biopsy confirmed the diagnosis.

287 **Idiopathic retroperitoneal fibrosis.** Section from retroperitoneal tissues showing an active phase with a heavy infiltrate of a mixture of chronic inflammatory cells (at the top of the picture) with some fibrosis (at the bottom). *(H&E × 160)*

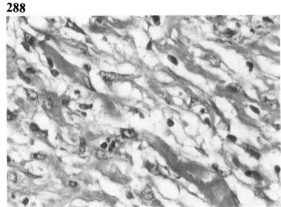

288 **Idiopathic retroperitoneal fibrosis.** Section showing more mature, dense fibrous tissue with little inflammatory cell infiltrate. *(H&E × 256)*

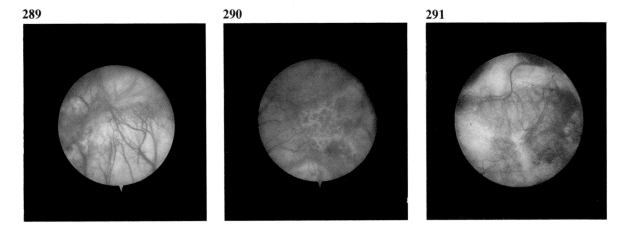

Cystitis

289 **Endoscopic changes in the bladder** show in the early stages the injected appearance of slightly engorged mucosal blood vessels.

290 **A patchy inflammation** will be seen with mild cystitis.

291 **A more severe form.**

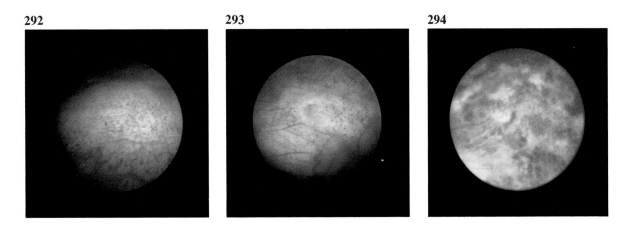

292 **Punctate haemorrhages** are noted.

293 **Inflammation around a ureteric orifice.**

294 **Florid acute cystitis.**

295 Cystourethritis may be accompanied by inflammatory polypi at the bladder neck. There is a variable degree of bladder neck inflammation.

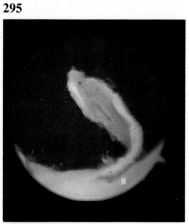

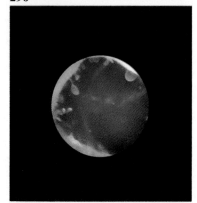

296 Shows the rarer polypi at the male bladder neck.

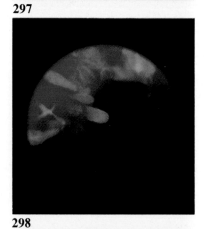

297 Florid posterior urethritis with polypi.

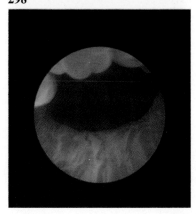

298 Prostatitis. In the male, prostatitis can occur with this characteristic appearance of an intensely red and oedematous bladder neck and prostatic urethral mucosa.

299 Acute cystitis. An oedematous mucosa with very congested blood vessels with red cells spilling out of the vessels where margination of neutrophil polymorphonuclear leucocytes is seen. This is basically an early vascular phase of the acute inflammatory reaction. Later in the process one of the elements of the reaction may predominate, giving a picture which may be described as bullous, fibrinous, purulent or haemorrhagic. *(H&E × 256)*

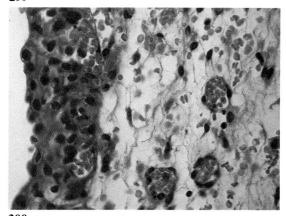
299

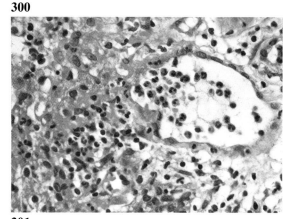
300

300 Acute cystitis. A severe acute inflammatory reaction. This is a cystitis induced by cyclophosphamide therapy. It becomes chronic leading to a small contracted bladder. *(H&E × 256)*

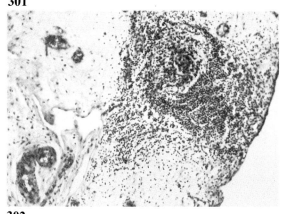
301

301 Chronic cystitis. An attenuated epithelium covering thickened connective tissue in which there is a heavy but patchy infiltrate of chronic inflammatory cells, mainly lymphocytes. *(H&E × 64)*

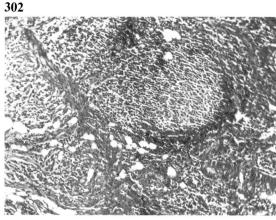
302

302 Chronic cystitis. Wall of the bladder with a heavy lymphoid infiltrate in which the aggregates of lymphoid cells have germinal centres. This pattern is often called follicular cystitis. *(H&E × 160)*

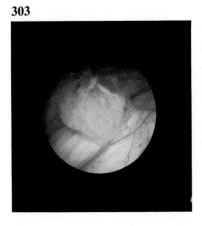 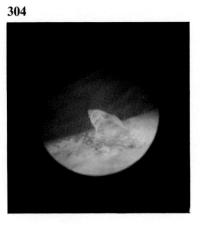 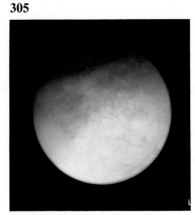

303 Fibromucous plaques. With more longstanding infection fibromucous plaques may be deposited on the urothelial surface.

304 Bladder bullae may also be noted. This process is entirely benign. Inflammatory proliferative conditions are also found in the bladder and include cystitis cystica and glandularis.

305 Cystitis cystica with clear cysts raised above the mucosa.

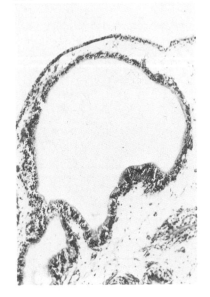

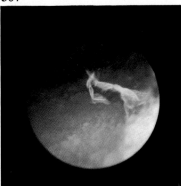

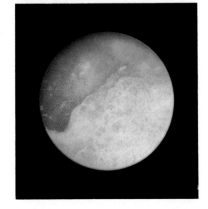

306 Cystitis cystica. Attenuated epithelium (at the top) is spread out over a cystically dilated cavity lined with transitional epithelium. A few chronic inflammatory cells are present in the connective tissue (see also **476**). *(H&E × 64)*

307 and 308 Cystitis glandularis shows more florid cystic changes, and the bladder may show a 'cobblestone' appearance.

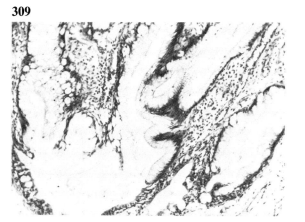

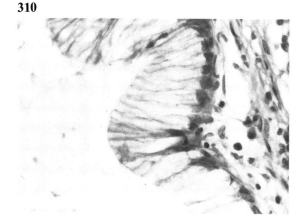

309 Cystitis glandularis. In the wall of the bladder there are cystic spaces lined mainly by tall columnar epithelium, which distinguishes this condition from cystitis cystica. *(H&E × 64)*

310 Cystitis glandularis. A higher magnification of × 85 showing the columnar epithelium, which is very different from the normal transitional epithelium. Adenocarcinoma may sometimes arise in this type of epithelium. *(H&E × 256)*

311 Squamous metaplasia of trigone. The well-demarcated white edge of squamous metaplasia of the trigone is entirely benign, presents itself in women, and probably has hormonal causes.

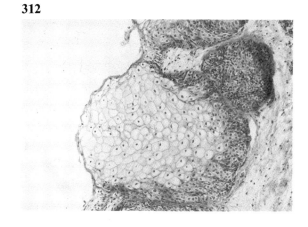

312 Squamous metaplasia of trigone. Bladder wall from the trigone where the normal transitional epithelium shows a squamoid maturation towards the surface, though it is not keratinising. *(H&E × 64)*

313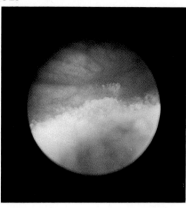

314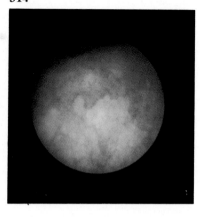

315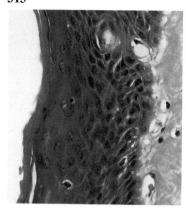

313 and 314. Another form of squamous metaplasia occurs with chronic irritation of the bladder and this more widespread form, which is shown, is often called leukoplakia. It is of more sinister significance because neoplasms can develop in such areas.

315 Leukoplakia. Section of bladder mucosa showing squamous epithelium which is keratinising. The epithelial cells show mild atypia and the underlying connective tissue shows some hyalinisation. Moist keratin appears as a white plaque on visual examination. Not all keratinising areas on mucosal surfaces are premalignant. *(H&E × 256)*

316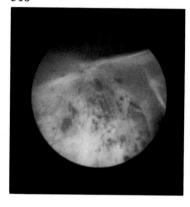

316 Interstitial cystitis, originally described in women by Hunner in 1915, is a chronic and painful irritable bladder syndrome, of unknown origin. The endoscopic appearance is characteristic with the radiate flare haemorrhages and ulcers in the bladder dome. Despite the sometimes localised ulcers, the changes are widespread in the bladder wall. The bladder may become progressively smaller and fibrotic.

317 Hunner's ulcer. Postmortem specimen of opened bladder showing classic red mucosal flares surrounding ulcerated area.

317a Hunner's ulcer. Section shows fibrosis and chronic inflammatory cells extending down into the muscle. *(H&E × 64)*

318 Hunner's ulcer. This section, in which fibrous tissue is stained green, shows the fibrosis in the wall which leads to a small contracted bladder. *(Trichrome × 64)*

317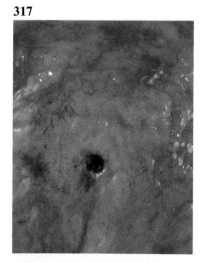

317a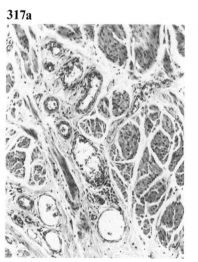

318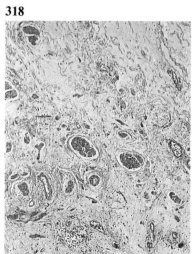

319

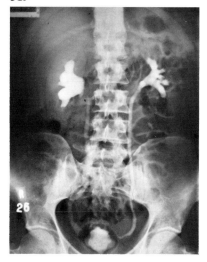

320

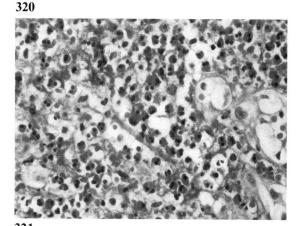

321

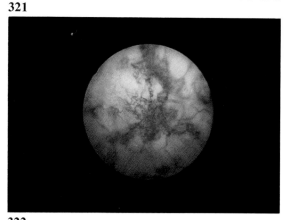

322

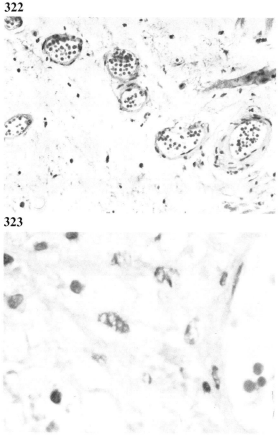

323

319 Eosinophilic cystitis. A rare form of inflammatory interstitial bladder disease is characterised by gross frequency, usually in men. The IVU shows the thickened bladder with the appearance of compression of the intramural ureters with obstruction of the upper tracts. Tuberculosis must always be excluded.

320 Eosinophilic cystitis. Section of bladder with a heavy infiltration of inflammatory cells in which the predominant cell is the eosinophil, with bi-lobed nuclei and bright eosinophilic, granular cytoplasm. *(H&E × 256)*

321 Irradiation cystitis is included as a form of 'inflammatory' cystitis. The endoscopic appearance is that of prominent vessels and blotchy haemorrhages interspersed with white atrophic areas of mucosa. This bleeds easily with bladder distention.

322 Irradiation cystitis. Telangiectatic blood vessels are prominent in this section of a post-irradiation bladder. *(H&E × 80)*

323 Irradiation cystitis. Fibrosis occurs in the wall of irradiated bladders and the fibroblasts often have an abnormal appearance. In this section the nuclei of fibro-blasts are vacuolated, a characteristic post-irradiation appearance. *(H&E × 256)*

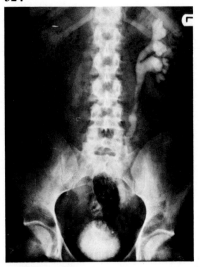

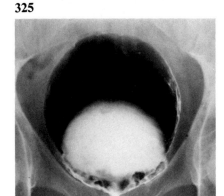

324 Malakoplakia. This rare granulomatous lesion, almost totally confined to the urinary tract, was first described by Michaelis and Guttmann in 1902. Occurring predominantly in women, it is probably a reaction to E. coli and usually presents with chronic cystitis, but can affect the upper tracts. In this IVU there is but minimal function on the right side and obstruction to the left ureter.

325 and 326 Double contrast cystography shows the vesical plaques of malakoplakia.

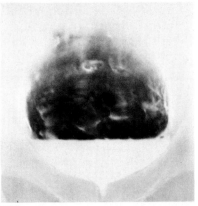

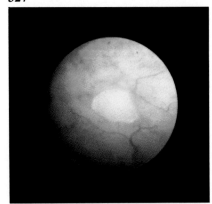

327 and 328 Endoscopic appearance of the soft yellow plaques.

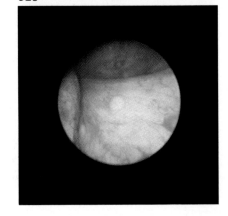

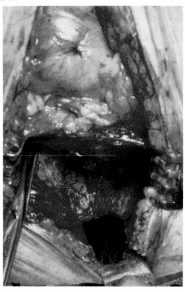 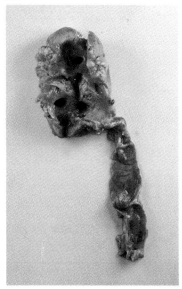 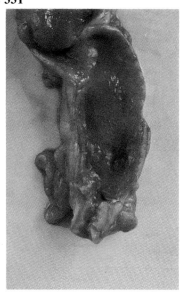

329   **Surgical appearance.** Plaques can also be observed at open cystotomy.

330 and 331   **The nephroureterectomy specimen** shows gross hydronephrosis and hydroureter due to the stricture of the lower ureter caused by malakoplakia.

332   **Malakoplakia.** Sheets of histiocytes and some neutrophilic polymorphonuclear leucocytes. In the histiocytes some of the blue staining bodies are nuclei (with a vesicular, predominantly oval appearance), but others appear as rather empty blue bodies, some laminated. The latter are Michaelis-Guttman bodies. *(H&E × 256)*

332

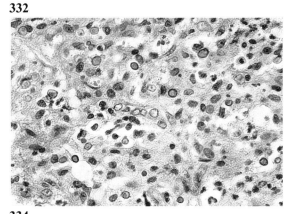

333   **Malakoplakia.** This stain demonstrates the calcium (black) which is present in Michaelis-Guttman bodies. *(von Kossa × 256)*

334   **Michaelis-Guttman body.** An electron micrograph of a histiocyte showing its nucleus (more or less centre field) and a calcified Michaelis-Guttman body in the upper part of the field on the left. They probably represent the end result of incomplete lysosomal digestion of engulfed E. coli.

333

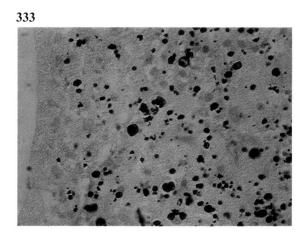

334

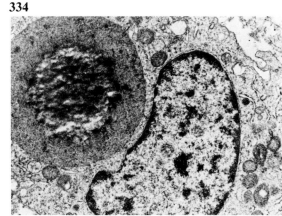

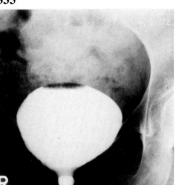
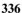

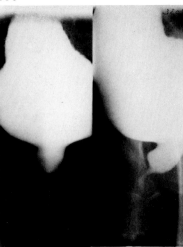

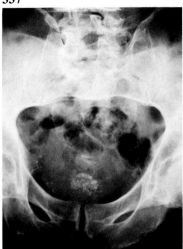

335 and 336   Inflammatory disease of the female urethra may be associated with urethral stenosis, seen in this MCU.

337   Chronic prostatitis in the male is usually abacterial but in the presence of prostatic calculi, chronic bacterial infection may occur. Chlamydia must also be excluded.

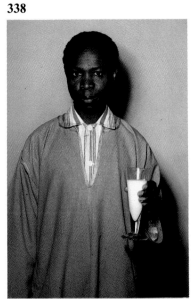

338   Chyluria. Milky urine as a result of the presence of chyle is rare except in patients from filarial-endemic areas. The parasite, Wuchereria bancrofti invades the lymphatics and causes an inflammatory reaction, which results in obstruction. The parasite is a nematode. Mature helminths live in connective tissue and lymphatics. The microfilariae are released into the bloodstream usually at night. A wide variety of symptoms result but those seen in urology usually result from lymphatic obstruction. Megalymphatics developing as a result may fistulate to the urinary tract and thus produce chyluria. Patient showing specimen of milky urine.

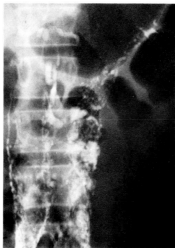
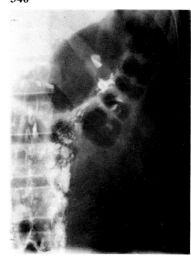

339 Chyluria. Lymphangiogram studies show dye tracking towards the region of the left kidney.

340 Chyluria. Later studies show the calyces well outlined confirming a fistula.

341 Chyluria. Where these fistulae occur in the kidney megalymphatics may be found in the renal pedicle at exploration.

342 Parasitic chyluria. Diagram of megalymphatics. Points of ligations are shown.

341

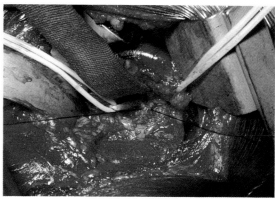

342

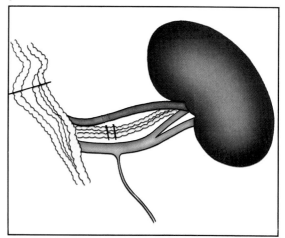

343 Chyluria. Patient with a specimen of clear urine after lymphatic ligation. Rarely the syndrome of chylous reflux in primary lymphoedema may produce chyluria as a result of obstruction both in the megalymphatic syndrome and in lymphatic deficiency.

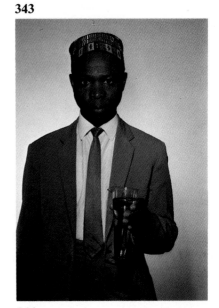

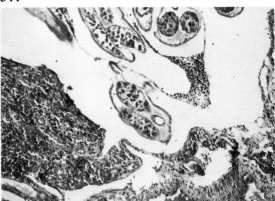

344 Wuchereria bancrofti. Section through adult worms (centre and upper field) with surrounding inflammatory reaction. *(H&E × 64)*

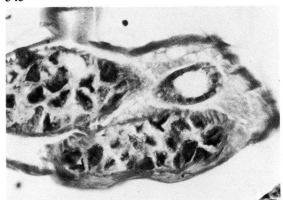

345 Wuchereria bancrofti. Higher magnification of section through an adult worm. *(H&E × 256)*

4 Tuberculosis

Genitourinary tuberculosis is one manifestation of a systemic disease which is caused by the vascular metatastic spread of the mycotuberculosis from a primary focus, usually in the lung. It is a disease seen less and less in the western world because of modern chemotherapy, but still poses many problems in the Third World countries. Semb (1953) pointed out the similarity between the pulmonary and renal lesion and emphasised they were two different aspects of the same disease, producing identical pathological changes.

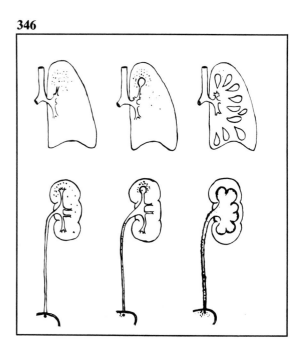

346 Semb diagrammatic portrayal of the similarity between the pulmonary and renal lesion. He suggested that the changes should be categorised into three groups.

	Kidney	Lung
Group 1	Medlar focus	Ghon focus
Group 2	Ulcerocavernous calyceal lesion	Pulmonary cavitation
Group 3	Extensive destruction of both the kidney and the lung	

It is important that any disease should be classified so that its progress can be accurately assessed and analysed.

347 New classification of genitourinary tuberculosis. The commonest presentation of genitourinary tuberculosis is of a young male with painless nocturia and increasing lack of energy which may or may not be accompanied by diurnal frequency. Dysuria is uncommon unless there is superimposed secondary infection; haematuria is only present in approximately 10 per cent of cases, and renal pain in 15 to 20 per cent. There are three important investigations – 1 Radiology, not only of the renal tract but also of the chest, which might show scarring indicative of an original primary focus. 2 Urinalysis looking especially for sterile pyuria, i.e. 20 cells per 1/6 HPF, which is present in over 70 per cent of cases. 3 Examination of three or more early morning specimens of urine for the isolation of mycobacterium tuberculosis and the mycobacterium bovis.

The organisms which cause tuberculosis are the mycobacterium tuberculosis and the mycobacterium bovis, both of which are acid and alcohol fast. Both these organisms show differences in morphology. The human strain is slender and may be slightly curved, and the bovine strain is straight and stubby and may occur singly or in pairs. Both these organisms are non-motile.

347

1 Kidney
   a) Tuberculous bacilluria or small calyceal lesion visible on a urogram
   b) Ulcerocavernous lesion
   c) Gross disease of the whole kidney
2 Kidneys, ureter and bladder with or without involvement of the external genitalia
3 Infection only involving the external genitalia

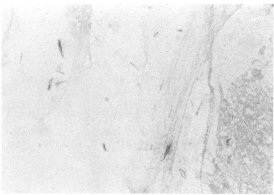

348 and 349 Mycobacterium tuberculosis (Zeihl-Nielsen stain). Both the mycobacterium tuberculosis and bovis are demonstrated by using a strong acting dye such as carbolfuchsin, with a counterstain such as methylene blue, as carried out in the Ziehl-Nielsen method. These two figures show mycobacterium tuberculosis which appear as red elongated rods. *(Ziehl-Nielsen × 640)*

349

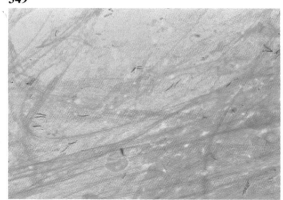

350

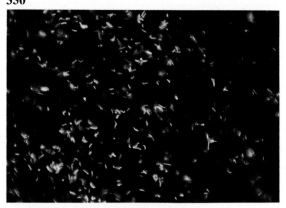

350 Mycobacterium tuberculosis (auramine rhodamine stain). This is used with fluorescent microscopy when the organisms show up as bright golden rods. *(Rhodamine auramine × 256)*

351

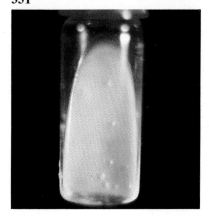

351 Mycobacterium tuberculosis, growing on Lowenstein-Jensen medium. The standard culture method for growing mycobacterium is on Lowenstein-Jensen medium with or without pyruvate. This figure shows a number of colonies which are whitish or buff coloured and discrete. Malachite green in the Lowenstein-Jensen medium not only helps to control contamination, but also serves to accentuate the buff colonies of the mycobacterium.

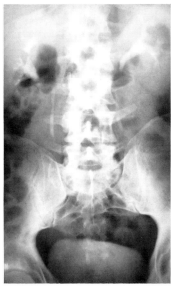
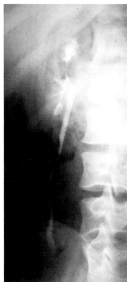

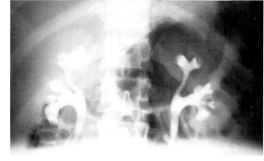

355

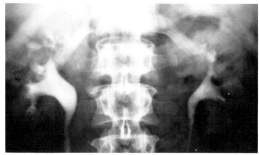

356

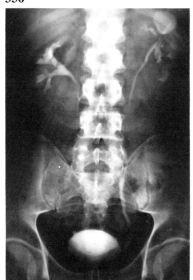

Intravenous urography (IVU)

The tuberculous lesions in the kidney as demonstrated by the IVU, vary from a small focus affecting only one calyx to total destruction. The initial lesion is in the parenchyma of the kidney, close to the glomeruli which spreads medially to involve the collecting system, producing tubercle bacilli in the urine. These lesions go on expanding until they produce the many different changes seen on the IVU.

Any tuberculous infection appears to be of two types – 1 A fulminating acute process with poor host resistance, which causes the ulcerocavernous lesion and destruction of renal tissue; 2 A less progressive type caused by a less virulent organism which together with a more effective host resistance causes the slowly growing fibrotic type of lesion.

352 IVU of a minor lesion affecting the upper pole of the right kidney. Note the disorganisation of the upper calyx.

353 Same lesion, oblique view. On this view the extent of the lesion is more easily seen.

354 IVU of a minor lesion of the upper pole of the right kidney, becoming more invasive. In this patient the disease has spread to affect more than one calyx, which have become irregular and deformed with papillary cavitation.

355 IVU of typical trifoliate lesion of the upper pole of the right kidney. This is a later lesion in which the disease has involved the neck of the calyx which then becomes constricted, resulting in classic cicatrical appearance.

356 IVU of ulcerocavernous disease. The disease has progressed still further and renal substance has been destroyed. Note that the damage is closely related to a calyx and that the cortical thickness remains unimpaired, but the cavity involves both renal tissue and the calyceal system.

357 IVU of solitary ulcerocavernous lesion in the middle calyx, a rare manifestation.

358 IVU of a more advanced middle calyceal lesion, only shown on retrograde pyelogram, an investigation now rarely required, because an IVU nearly always supplies all the necessary information.

359 IVU of a combined stenosing lesion of the middle calyx, with destructive cavitation changes in the lower pole.

357

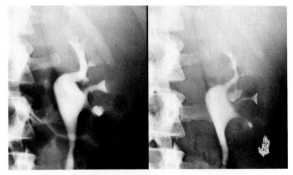

358

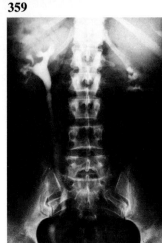

359

360 IVU of an example of the disease involving multiple calyces but showing minimal parenchymal damage, again emphasising that cortical involvement is a very late phenomenon.

361 IVU of another example of a more advanced disease involving multiple calyces. This shows more parenchymal damage, but the function is good. This type of lesion is usually of many years duration and is caused by organisms of low virulence.

360

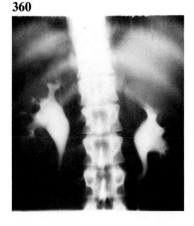

361

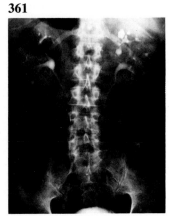

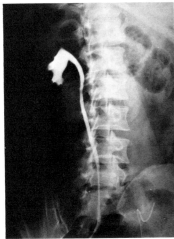

362

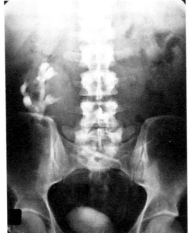

363

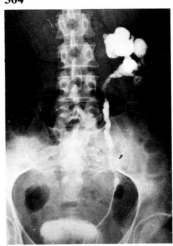

364

362 IVU of extensive low-grade disease causing fibrosis of the calyceal stem so that the area of the kidney which drains into the diseased calyceal system ceases to function, and on urography gives the typical 'cut off' appearance.

363 IVU of a moderate lesion affecting one half of a horseshoe kidney. Congenital abnormal kidneys are rarely affected by the mycobacterium, but infection can occur.

364 IVU of an example of unilateral extensive disease.

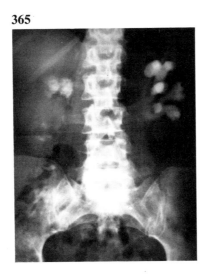

365

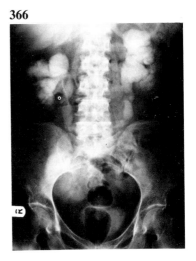

366

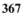

365 and 366 IVU of examples of bilateral extensive disease. In the type of lesion shown in **364**, **365** and **366** the disease has progressed to destroy a large part of functioning renal tissue; the urographic appearances reveal a disorganised pelviureteric system with cavities in the renal parenchyma.

Macroscopic appearance

367 Gross renal tuberculosis, showing almost complete destruction of renal tissue. The cortex is thinned and numerous cavities are present. This is the end result of longstanding disease.

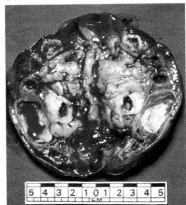

367

368

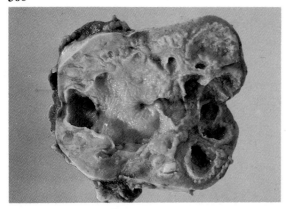

368 Renal tuberculosis. A different type of lesion demonstrating a smaller kidney, fewer cavities, almost total cortical destruction with numerous cortical abscesses.

369a Complete destruction of kidney by tuberculosis.

369b Radiograph shows calcification in this caseous pyonephrosis.

Renal tuberculosis

Histology

370 Renal tuberculosis. In the bottom righthand corner of the picture is a glomerulus. In the centre and upper lefthand side of the picture is a giant-cell granuloma. This is composed of a central zone of histiocytic cells (which are derived from monocytes in the blood), some of which have become epithelioid in appearance (i.e. their plentiful cytoplasm has become eosinophilic and they resemble squamous cells). Others have fused to form a multinucleate giant cell which has its nuclei arranged around the periphery of the cell (i.e. it is a Langhan's type giant cell). Around the periphery of the granuloma there are lymphocytes and plasma cells. This granuloma is in the cortex of the kidney; it has not yet undergone the central necrosis which is seen as caseation in older granulomas. *(H&E × 160)*

371 Renal tuberculosis. In the medulla there is widespread infiltration with chronic inflammatory cells and the tubules are being destroyed. There is necrosis and the papilla is undergoing necrosis and has a ragged edge (on the lefthand side of the picture). *(H&E × 160)*

369a

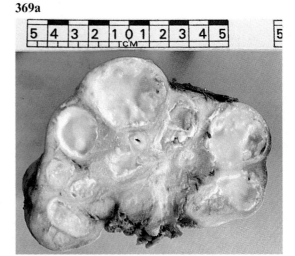

369b

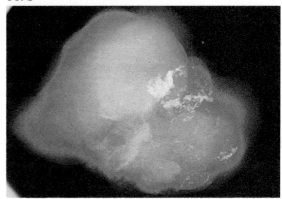

370

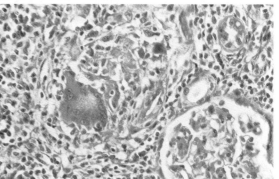

371

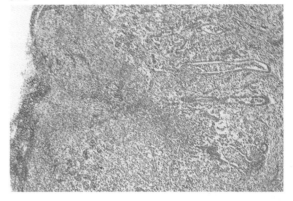

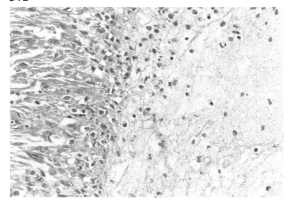

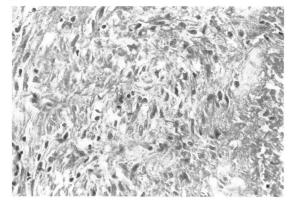

372 Renal tuberculosis. A later stage in granulomatous inflammation. The histiocytic cells are seen to be surrounding a pale area of caseous necrosis. Some lymphocytes and occasional polymorphs are also present at the junction of these two zones. *(H&E × 160)*

373 Renal tuberculosis. A longstanding lesion. Some necrosis is evident (at the righthand side of the picture), but in most of the field there is plentiful eosinophilic collagen being laid down by the fibroblasts which are replacing the inflammatory cells. This fibrosis is frequently seen around old tuberculous lesions and it often calcifies.

Occasionally renal tuberculosis affects one half of a duplex system and very rarely both moieties. *(H&E × 160)*

374 IVU of extensive renal tuberculosis involving only one moiety of a bifid kidney. It is an interesting fact that once the diseased moiety is removed, the other moiety never gets infected.

374

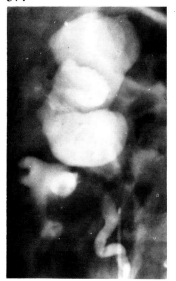

375

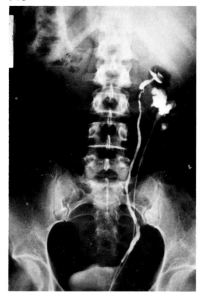

375 IVU of extensive renal tuberculosis involving only one moiety of a bifid kidney.

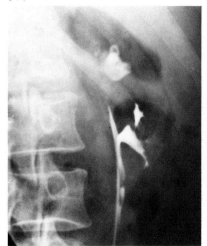

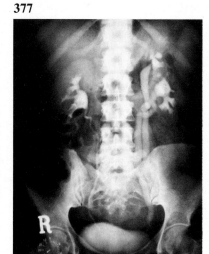

376 IVU of a lateral view which may outline the lesion in greater detail.

377 IVU of examples of renal tuberculosis affecting both moieties of a duplex kidney, a very rare manifestation.

Calcification

Calcification is becoming an important clinical finding because 50 per cent of patients have a calcified lesion somewhere in the renal tract when first seen. When a lesion is present, patients should have the same investigations as those presenting with calculi in the renal tract. The calcified lesion varies from a small discrete area in the kidney to involvement of all parts of the urinary system. It appears to be of two types, progressive and static, hence the danger and the importance of following up patients with calcification for an indefinite period, because it is impossible to tell whether it will worsen or remain unchanged for years.

378 **379** **380**

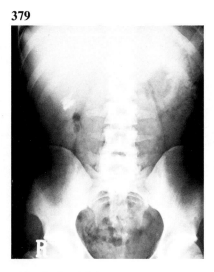

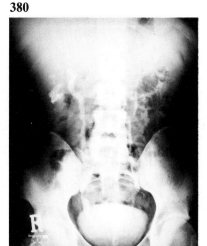

378 Calcification: small discrete renal calculus (plain urogram). A lesion which is impossible to distinguish from a solitary renal calculus until mycobacterium is isolated from the urine.

379 and 380 Calcification: larger area (plain urogram and IVU). A progressive type which usually involves either the upper or lower pole.

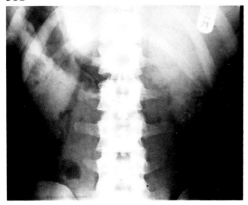

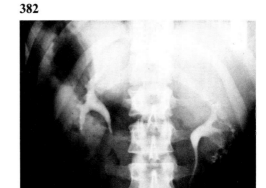

381 and 382   Calcification: another larger area (plain and IVU). This is an unusual presentation, because it simulates nephrocalcinosis with minimal parenchymal damage, a lesion which cannot be confirmed until mycobacterium is isolated from the urine.

383

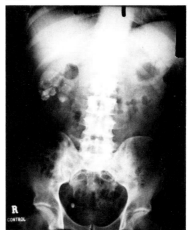

383 and 384   Calcification affecting upper pole (plain and IVU). This is a static type, which has been present for about 20 years without alteration. Note the satisfactory function of the remaining parts of the kidney.

384

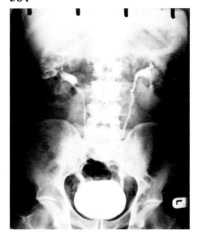

385 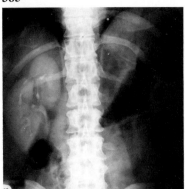 **386** 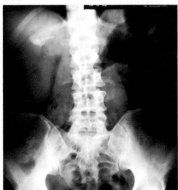 **387**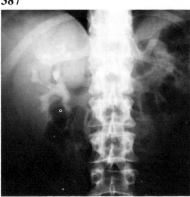

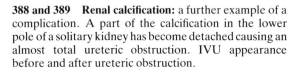

385, 386 and 387 A progressive type of calcification affecting the upper pole of a solitary kidney. **385** shows minimal calcification with scarring, **386** and **387** show the direct and intravenous urographic appearance one year later.

388 and 389 Renal calcification: a further example of a complication. A part of the calcification in the lower pole of a solitary kidney has become detached causing an almost total ureteric obstruction. IVU appearance before and after ureteric obstruction.

Progressive calcification can spread slowly and insidiously and take many years to destroy the kidney. This is an example of what can happen if patients with calcification are not supervised properly. This patient had a cavernotomy for the calcified lesion in the lower pole of the left kidney, but the pathology in the right kidney was not considered severe.

388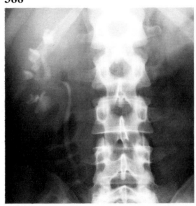

389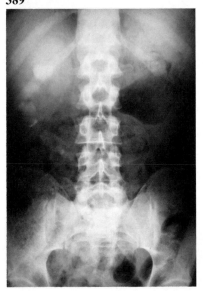

390   IVU of condition before cavernotomy.

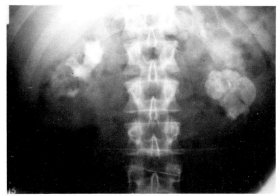

390

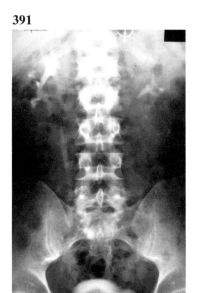

391

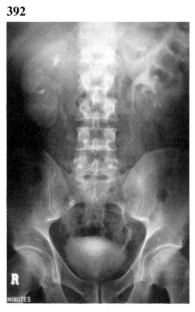

392

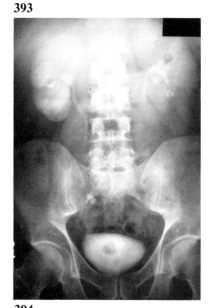

393

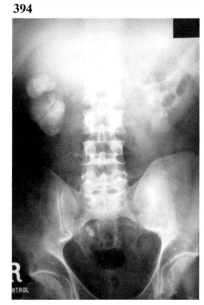

394

391   One year later, diffuse calcification in the lower pole of the right kidney.

392   One year later, the calcification is denser.

393   One year later, further increase in the spread and density of the calcification.

394   Calcification: one year later. Two-thirds of the kidney has been destroyed by slow progressive calcification. The mycobacterium is never isolated from these patients. On histological examination the section shows chronic pyelonephritis with diffuse parenchymal calcification.

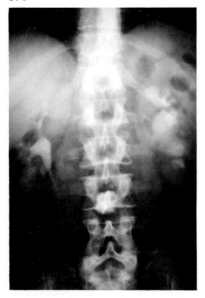

395

395 Calcification in the upper pole with active disease and hydronephrosis.

396 Calcification with active caseating disease. In this resected upper pole specimen the calcification is shown in the middle of an area in which the renal parenchyma has been destroyed. This is the progressive type; in this type of lesion a selective renal arteriogram may help to decide the amount of kidney to be excised, because invariably more renal damage is present than is shown in an IVU.

397 Multiple calculi in a tuberculous kidney (plain urogram).

398 Multiple calculi with hydronephrosis (plain urogram).

The calcified kidney may be contracted and situated over the psoas muscle. In this type of case it may be difficult to differentiate it from a calcified psoas abscess, without an IVU. However, if the latter is the cause of the calcification, destructive changes in the vertebrae should be present. It is essential to xray the thoracic as well as the dorsal spine, because the abscess may track down from the thoracic region before entering the sheath of the psoas muscle.

396

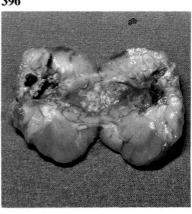

397

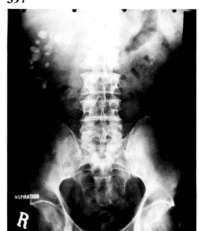

398

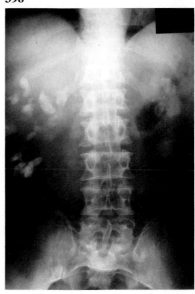

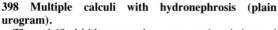

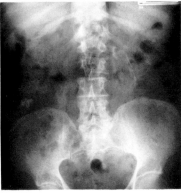

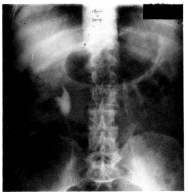

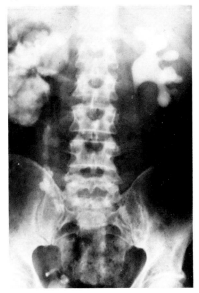

399   Plain film of a calcified shadow over the left psoas muscle.

400   An IVU which reveals a non-functioning left kidney.

401   Calcification involving one kidney, ureter, seminal vesicles and the prostate (plain urogram).

Tuberculosis of the ureter

Tuberculosis which affects the ureter can cause strictures at the pelviureteric junction, in the middle third of the ureter and at the uretervesical junction. The commonest site is the ureterovesical junction.

402   IVU of a stricture forming at the pelviureteric junction. This is a rare manifestation because the combination of an acute virulent infection with an obstruction at the pelviureteric junction destroys the kidney before treatment can be started. Nevertheless, when diagnosed, treatment must be aggressive to relieve the obstruction.

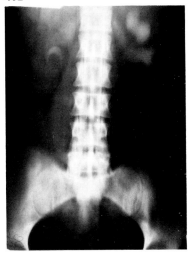

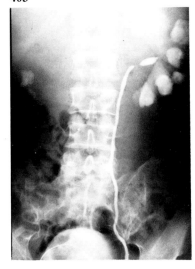

403   Two strictures. Another rare manifestation involving the pelvis, causing obstruction of the pelvicalyceal junction and all the calyceal stems. This condition poses great problems in treatment especially if the kidney is solitary.

Strictures of the middle third of the ureter are very rare, but if seen early enough can be effectively treated.

404

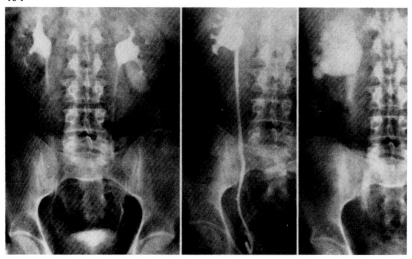

405

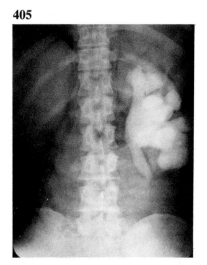

406

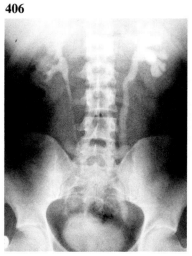

407

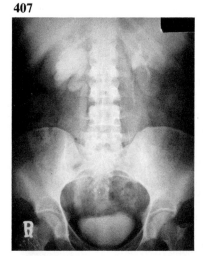

408

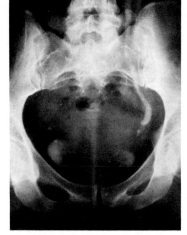

404   IVU of stricture of the middle third of the ureter, treated by prolonged ureteric catheterisation with a silastic tube.

405   IVU of a stricture of the upper third of the ureter with hydronephrosis. A very rare manifestation.

Strictures of the lower end of the ureter can be caused by oedema or fibrosis.

406   IVU of early stricture of the lower end of the ureter, with commencing dilatation of the whole of the upper urinary tract.

407   IVU of more advanced stricture of the lower end of the ureter in which the hydronephrosis is more pronounced.

408   IVU of stricture of the lower end of a bifid system.

Strictures may be multiple, but this is another rare manifestation. It is more usual to find the whole of the ureter replaced by fibrous tissue.

409

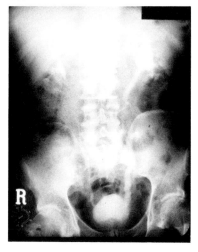

410

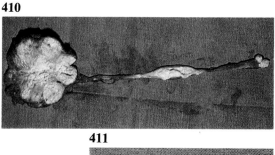

411

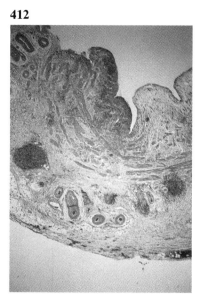

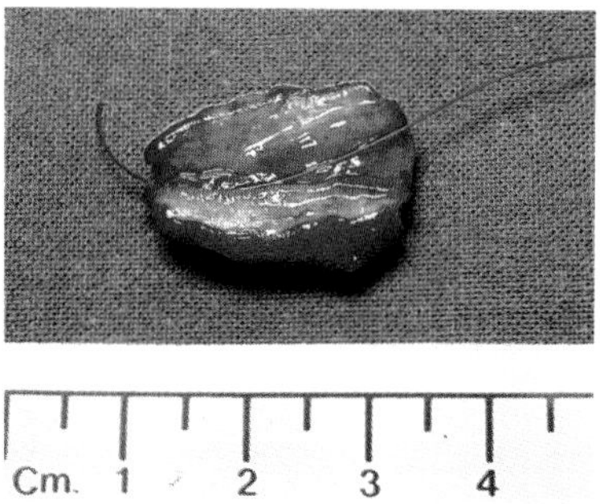

409 IVU of stricture at the pelviureteric junction and at the ureterovesical junction.

410 A kidney completely destroyed by a combination of strictures at the pelviureteric junction, the mid third of the ureter and the ureterovesical junction.

411 Specimen of excised ureterovesical stricture, showing fibrosis, oedema and narrow lumen. The disease in this patient has advanced far beyond the reach of conservative treatment.

412

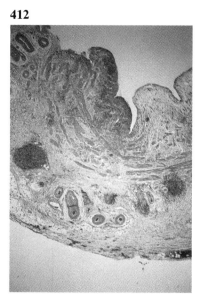

413

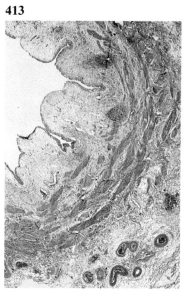

414

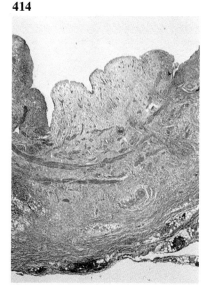

412 Microscopic appearance of 411. Wall of the ureter showing chronic inflammatory cells extending right through the wall, with fibrosis occurring in all coats. The mucosa is oedematous. The underlying bands of muscle, stained dark pink, are separated and the inflammatory cells (blue) are scattered through the wall and aggregated into groups.

413 Histological appearance of the ureter stained with trichrome, showing extensive fibrous infiltration.

414 Section from the same ureter stained with trichrome which stains the fibrous tissue green.

415 Fibrous tissue separating the muscle bands and involving the mucosa. Lymphoid aggregates are seen but there are no granulomata.

A very rare finding is a calcified stricture at the lower end of the ureter causing almost complete obstruction.

416   A plain film of such a ureter.

417   IVU showing hydronephrosis and poor renal function.

418   Specimen showing calcification and a thickened fibrous ureter.

415

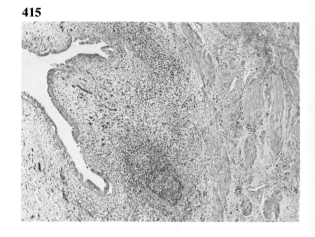

416

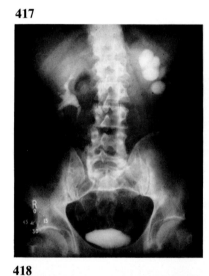

417

418

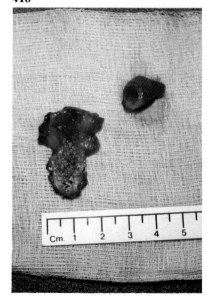

419   **420**   **421**

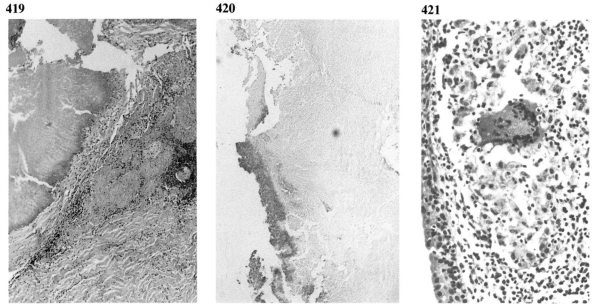

419 Histological appearance of calcified area after total decalcification, showing caseous material (upper lefthand side of field).

420 Ziehl-Nielsen of amorphous tissue after treatment showing clumps of degenerate bacilli.

421 Tuberculous granuloma in the ureter.

Endoscopy

Tuberculous cystitis presents in many ways, but always starts with a mild inflammation around a tuberculous orifice. It can spread and involve the whole bladder producing an intense diffuse cystitis.

422 Tuberculous cystitis: a mild infection. The orifice is mildly oedematous and beginning to gape. Every case of tuberculous cystitis starts at a ureteric orifice.

423 Tuberculous cystitis. If the infection is more severe, the orifice becomes acutely inflamed and the inflammation spreads to the bladder.

424 Tuberculous cystitis. As the infection develops profuse granulations appear and the orifice cannot be seen.

422

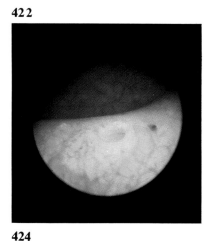

423

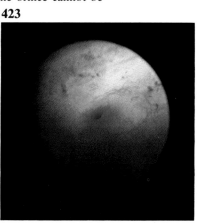

424

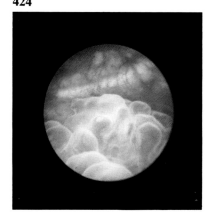

425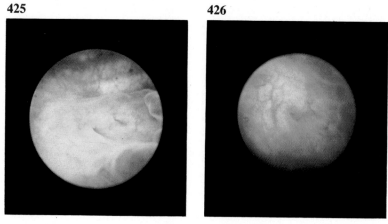

427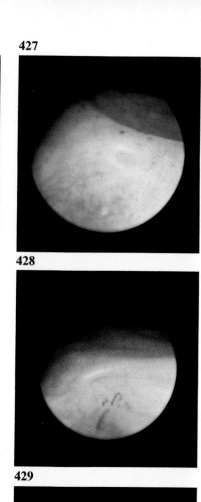

425 Tuberculous cystitis. As healing progresses the granulations disappear and the orifice can then be seen.

Ultimately the orifice can almost return to normal but is usually rigid, (**426**), or appears pale (**427**), hooded (**428**) and withdrawn (**429**).

430 Small golf-hole ureter. It is irregular and the surrounding mucus membrane is pale and atrophic.

428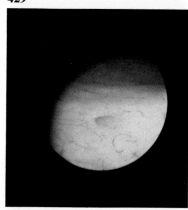

429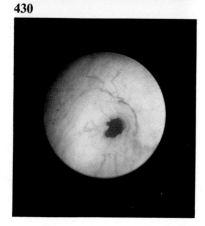

430

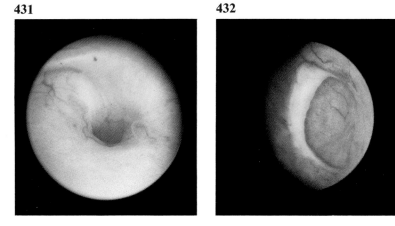 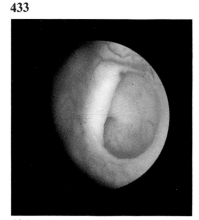

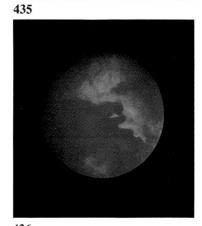

434

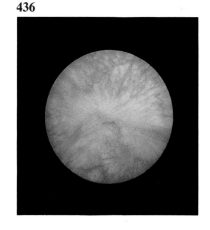

431   **Golf-hole ureter** which is a rigid healed orifice.

432   **Golf-hole ureter.** In a severe infection granulations completely cover the ureteric orifice so that it cannot be seen. Once healing begins, the granulation slowly disappears leaving an inflamed oedematous orifice. In this type of case, which is responding rapidly to modern chemotherapy, the orifice ultimately looks scarred and occasionally hooded.

In the more longstanding case the ureter becomes withdrawn, producing the classic golf-hole appearance. This can be clearcut or surrounded by a hood of fibrous tissue with the orifice visible in the floor of a superficial diverticulum.

433   **Golf-hole ureter** seen in the floor of a false diverticulum.

434   **Acute tuberculous ulcer** showing central slough.

435   **Bladder tuberculosis.** Once the tuberculous disease has spread to the bladder, it can cause ulceration or a diffuse tuberculous cystitis.

436   **Healed cystitis scar.** When the cystitis heals it produces a scar often in stellate form and very similar to that of a Hunner's ulcer.

435

436

Histology

437 Section of bladder wall showing a giant-cell granuloma in the connective tissue, beneath the transitional cell epithelium.

In a severe infection the disease can involve the kidney, ureter, bladder, epididymes and even the urethra.

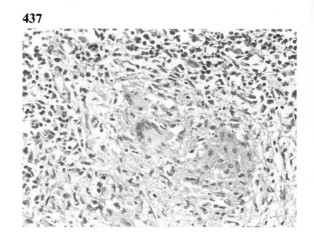

437

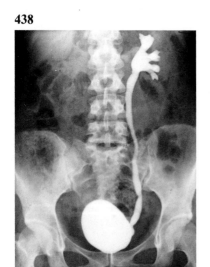

438

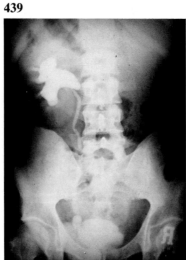

439

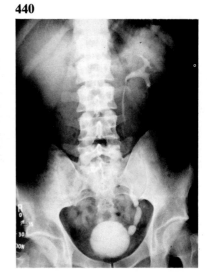

440

438 IVU of tuberculous cystitis with stricture at the lower end of the ureter, showing a contracted bladder.

439 IVU of advanced tuberculous cystitis with stricture at the lower end of the ureter, showing a contracted bladder.

440 IVU showing early tuberculous cystitis and an early ureteric stricture in which the urographic appearance of the kidney is still normal.

441

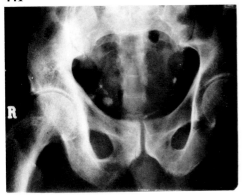

442

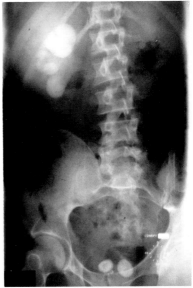

Tuberculosis of the seminal vesicles

Tuberculosis of the seminal vesicles is rare and is nearly always associated with tuberculous prostatitis and epididymitis; when the acute phase heals calcification is common.

441   Plain film of calcification in the seminal vesicles.

443

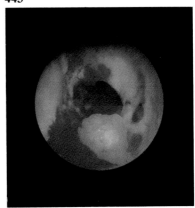

Tuberculous prostatitis

This condition occurs especially with tuberculosis of the epididymis. It often contains calculi.

442   IVU of calculi in the prostate with a small contracted bladder and hydronephrosis of a solitary kidney.

443   Endoscopic view of a tuberculous prostatitis showing the cavity from which the calculus has been extruded.

444

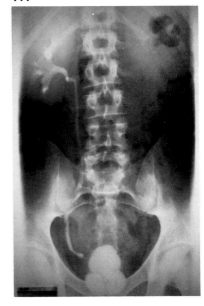

444   IVU of large prostatic cavities caused by destruction of the prostate.

445

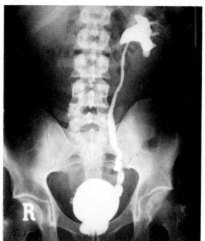

446

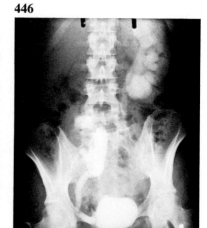

447

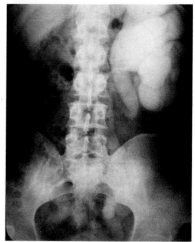

Generalised tuberculosis of the urinary tract

On rare occasions the infection may involve all parts of the genitourinary tract and pose severe problems in management.

445 IVU of tuberculous cystitis combined with a stricture at the lower end of the ureter, and tuberculous prostatic cavitation.

446 Tuberculous left kidney, tuberculous bladder and tuberculous right ectopic kidney.

447 Severe renal TB of a solitary kidney with ureteric reflex and a small contracted bladder.

448 Severe left renal TB with small contracted bladder and early stricture of the right ureter.

448

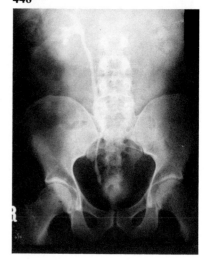

449

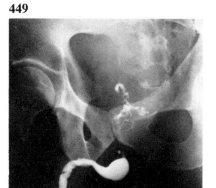

450

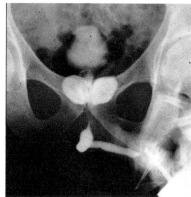

451

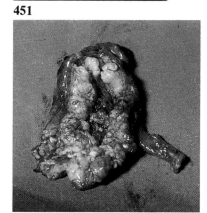

Urethral stricture

Tuberculous urethral stricture is rare and once the acute infection is under control it should be managed the same way as any other urethral stricture. On urography it cannot be distinguished from any other urethral stricture.

449 Ascending urethrogram of tuberculous urethral stricture.

450 Ascending urethrogram of tuberculous urethral stricture associated with a small contracted bladder, prostatic cavitation and a perineal fistula.

Tuberculous epididymitis is a common presenting sign and patients first complain of a painful scrotal swelling; usually there is no disturbance of micturition.

451 Tuberculous epididymitis.

452 Tuberculous epididymitis with a skin sinus.

453 Tuberculous epididymitis involving the testis, which occurs in five per cent of cases of tuberculous epididymitis.

452

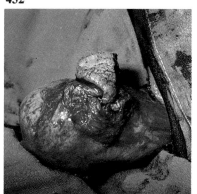

453

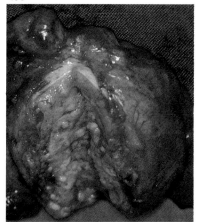

5 Schistosomiasis (bilharziasis) of the genitourinary system

Bilharziasis is a disease found in many parts of the world. However, it is mainly endemic in the greater part of Africa. The main species causing disease in man are S. Haematobium which predominantly affects the urinary tract and S. Mansoni and S. Japonicum which cause intestinal disease. Schistosoma Haematobium is a trematode. The adult male is 10 to 15 mm long and 2 mm broad. It has two suckers anteriorly. Its body is irregularly covered with round projections, which together with the suckers help the worm to anchor itself to the venous wall of the host. The female is 8 to 17 mm long and 1 mm wide and lies enclosed in the gynaecophoric canal of the male schistosoma.

454 Egg in the urine. The eggs are oval, about 120 mm in length and the shell has a distinct terminal spine. S. Mansoni has a subterminal spine, and the embryo is visible within. When the infected urine becomes diluted on being mixed with water, the shell swells and bursts and a ciliated embryo or miracidium escapes.

455 Ciliated miracidium. The miracidium swims actively searching for the intermediate hosts. The Bulinus contortus, a fresh-water snail, which when encountered is penetrated by the miracidia which eventually reach the liver where the develop into cercariae, forming multiple hepatic sporocysts.

456 Bulinus contortus. In about a month the snail dies, the ovocysts rupture and discharge thousands of cerceriae into the water.

457 Bulinus contortus discharging cercariae.

454

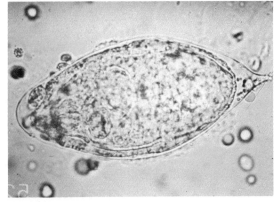

455

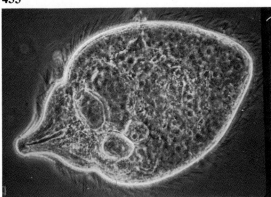

456

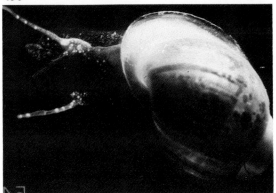

457

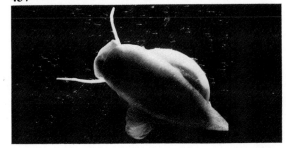

458 **Cercariae.** The cercaria is 2 mm long with a pear-shaped head and a bifid tail. They reach their definitive host, usually man, to infect him chiefly through the skin but also through the mucus membrane of the mouth and pharynx. The cerceria leaves its tail during penetration of the skin.

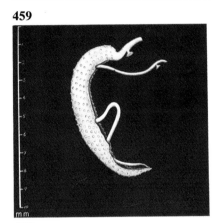

459 **Male worm with female in the gynaecophoric canal.**

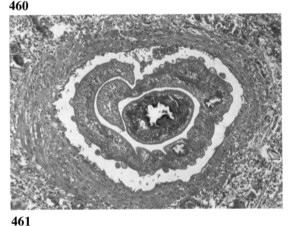

460 **Adult schistosomes.** The female lies enfolded in the gynaecophoric grooves of the male. They are both inside a small vein in the bladder wall. Some eggs and inflammation are seen in the surrounding tissues. *(H&E × 80)*

461 **Eggs in perivenous tissue.** These elicit an inflammatory reaction which may be very variable in its pattern. *(Periodic acid Schiff × 256)*

462   **463**   **464**

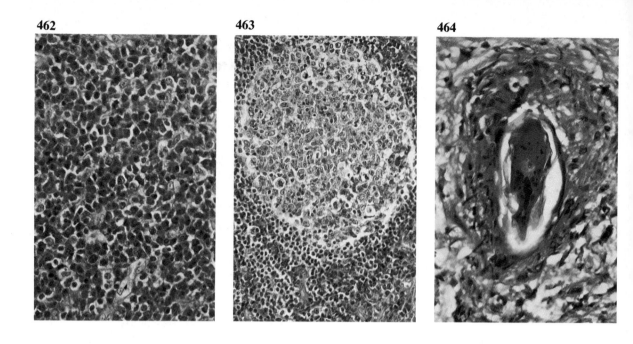

462 Schistosomiasis. Inflammation in the bladder wall. Here there is a very heavy infiltrate of eosinophils, with other inflammatory cells. *(H&E × 256)*

463 Schistosomiasis. Inflammation in the bladder wall. Occasionally lymphoid follicles with reactive centres form. *(H&E × 160)*

464 Schistosomiasis. Inflammation in the bladder wall showing some histiocytes surrounding an ovum. Fibrosis is present around the histiocytes. *(H&E × 256)*

465 Detailed schematic drawing of the life cycle of S. Haematobium as it affects man.

In the bladder the area which appears to be the portal of entry of bilharzia is known as the 'Magarr' which is the Arabic word for the milky way. This Magarr area extends from the right side of the bladder below the air bubble to cross the midline to the left side of the bladder where it assumes a more or less vertical direction which it maintains to about 3.5 cm above and to the left of the left ureteric orifice. Then it crosses the midline again to end about 2.5 cm to the right and above the right ureteric orifice. The Magarr area is at the junction of the fixed and mobile part of the bladder and it is at the junction of the part that is richly supplied with blood, the posterior and superior wall which is supplied by only one vessel the superior vesical artery. In the bladder during the early stages of bilharzial infestation the bladder looks as if it is affected with patchy congested areas that is acute mucosal patchy hyperaemia.

465

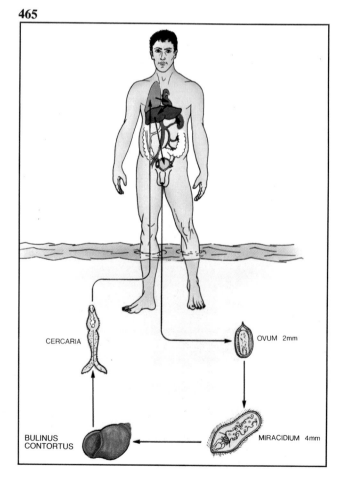

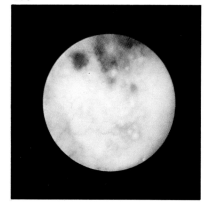

466 and 467 Cystoscopic appearance of the earliest acute bilharzial lesions in the bladder.

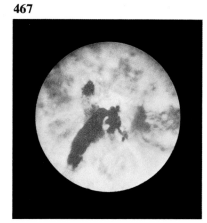

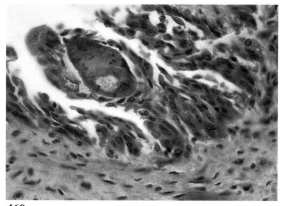

468 Bladder mucosa showing egg of schistosomiasis passing through the epithelium into the bladder lumen. *(H&E × 256)*

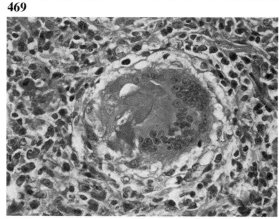

469 Bladder wall showing granuloma formation in response to the presence of eggs. Some of the histiocytes have fused to form a multinucleate giant cell. *(H&E × 256)*

470 Bladder wall showing dead ova with very little inflammatory reaction. The pink staining material is fibrous tissue. This would appear as a sandy patch on endoscopy. *(H&E × 160)*

470

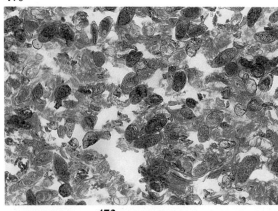

471

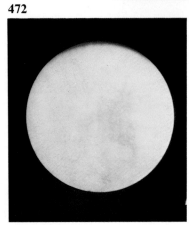

472

473

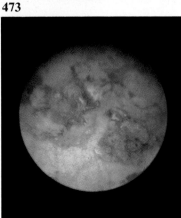

474

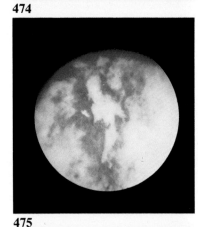

475

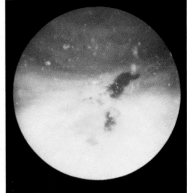

471 A sandy patch. This is caused by a mucosal reaction to the submucosal ova deposition in which whole layers of epithelium, except the basement membrane, are shed. The ova appear as packed sand under water and the areas are pale brown. Dead and calcified ova are deposited under wider areas of the mucosa and look as white as sheets.

472 Ground-glass mucosa. On other occasions the bladder mucosa can ulcerate and become infected.

473 Septic bilharzial ulcers. Rest of the vesical mucosa shows signs of inflammation.

474 Chronic superficial ulcer. Larger than the acute one, irregular edges, a pale anaemic floor surrounded by congested hyperaemia mucous membrane.

475 Chronic deep ulcer. Bilharzial tubercles on top, ground-glass mucosa below.

476 Cystitis cystica shows cystic spaces lined with transitional epithelium and showing inflammation. Occasionally the epithelium shows a glandular metaplasia and the condition is then called 'cystitis glandularis'. *(H&E × 160)*

476

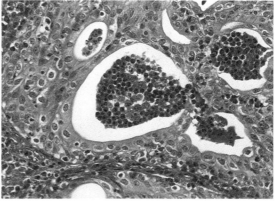

477 Chronic deep ulcer. Bilharzial tubercles above, ground-glass mucosa below. Ulcers show complete denudation of the mucosa including the basement membrane. The base of this lesion comprises granulation or fibrous tissue according to the stage of the ulcer, which may be acute or chronic Chronic ulcers may be superficial, deep, or stellate. Bilharzial ulcers never turn malignant.

The bladder mucosa may react more actively producing hyperplastic lesions such as cystitis cystica, cystitis glanularis, bilharzia polypi or malignant neoplasms.

477

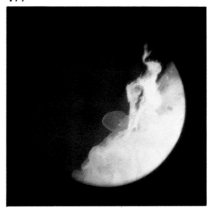

478 Bladder schistosomiasis. This bladder shows marked thickening, with the mucosa thrown up into polypoid folds.

478

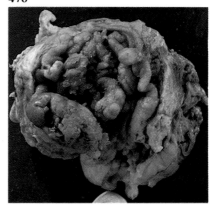

479a Bladder schistosomiasis. Section through the wall of **478** showing the mucosa with polyp formation. The epithelium is hyperplastic and covers cores of connective tissue. No neoplasm was present despite its florid appearances. *(H&E original section life size)*

479b Bladder schistosomiasis. Similar section to **479** but stained with a trichrome to show the fibrous tissue (green). *(Trichrome × 3)*

Radiologically these two conditions show as filling defects on urograms. When urinary crystalloids are deposited on the ruptured cysts, they appear as calcified shadows on plain xray.

479a

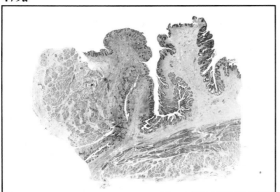

479b

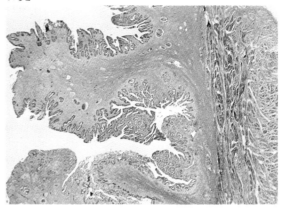

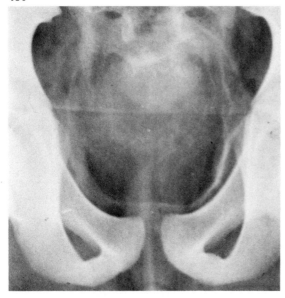

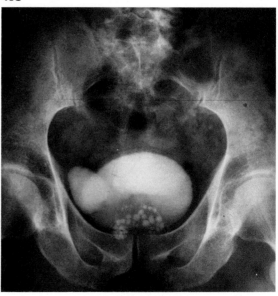

Bilharzial affection of the muscle layer of the bladder passes into three stages 1 Irritable bladder; 2 Weak bladder; 3 Contracted bladder.

480   IVU of bilharzial calcification of the bladder wall. The bladder is distended its upper border which has reached the sacroiliac joint. The stage of irritable bladder is before the stage of acute fibrosis. The muscle wall may be hypertrophied or at least spastic in the irritative phase of acite infiltration. The bladder is then thicker in its wall and may produce temporary pressure on the intravesical ureter, while the ureter itself continuing to contract may cause non-calcular renal colic or temporary back pressure on the upper parts of the ureter or even the kidney.

In the weak stage a mild fibrosis of the muscle will interfere with the power of contractility of the bladder. When fibrosis proceeds further it produces dilatation and thinning of the wall with the formation of a retrotrigonal pouch.

482   Endoscopic view of bladder-neck fibrosis. The disease may affect the Magarr line and produce a bipartite bladder or it may affect the whole organ causing a contracted bladder.

483   Cystogram showing a severely contracted bladder. The bladder may go from the normal to the hypertrophic, thick-walled state, then dilate again to retrieve its normal size, proceeding further to the dilated, atonic bladder only to recontract again, even to the useless scarred, non-contractile contracted bladder.

Calcification is a classical finding in longstanding bilharzial disease of the urinary tract. Not only the bladder and bladder-neck but also ureters may be involved.

481   Bladder-neck obstruction with diverticulum in the right lateral wall and multiple calculi in the retrotrigonal pouch. This either alone or together with an associated bladder-neck fibrosis resembles an elevated bladder neck. This may resolve under treatment. Or this may proceed further to a stage where one can find residual urine consequent upon dynamic atony as well as stenosis of the bladder neck. Finally contraction of the fibrous tissue commonly occurs and may be localised in the bladder-neck, giving the syndrome of bladder-neck fibrosis.

482

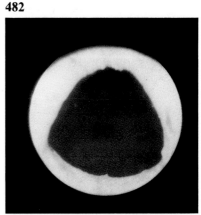

483

484 **Carcinoma of the bladder** occurs in association with schistosomiasis. About two-thirds of the carcinomas are of squamous type and may be related to squamous metaplasia occurring with the inflammation. About a quarter are transitional in type, while the remainder are adenocarcinomas. This section shows a squamous carcinoma with some associated eggs. *(H&E × 160)*

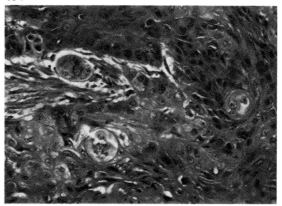

Radiological appearance of bilharzial bladder

485 **Plain xray of bilharzial calcified contracted bladder.**

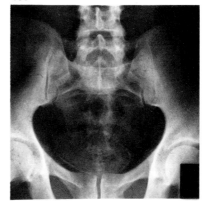

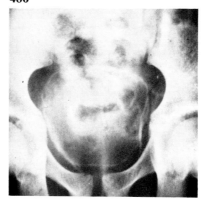

486 **Plain xray of laminated calcification of bilharzial bladder**, which also shows calcified dilated ureters, with ureteritis calcinosa (calcified ureteritis cystica). An elevated and calcified base of bladder, typical of bilharzial bladder-neck fibrosis, is also seen.

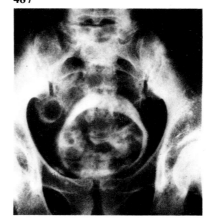

487 **Plain xray of a more advanced case of linear calcification of a dilated bladder** with calcified base of bilharzial bladder-neck fibrosis.

488a **Plain xray showing disappearance of calcification on left side of the bladder** resulting from carcinoma of the bladder.

488b **IVU showing the line of calcification on the left side which is destroyed by the tumour tissue.**

  Next to cystoscopy, as an important means of studying the pathology of vesical bilharziasis, comes radiography. Plain xray hardly reveals any bilharzial lesions before calcification. The appearance depends on the severity of calcification and density of fibrosis in the bladder wall. In mild cases, linear shadows of calcification of the bladder wall are visible. In more advanced cases, laminated calcification of the bladder wall is present. In severe cases, the vesical shadow forms a small circle or sphere, and the cavity of the bladder is being filled up with irregular opacities.
  In malignancy, distortion and dissolution of calcification can occur.

488a

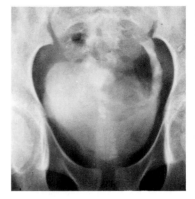

488b

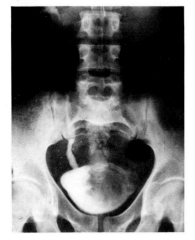

489

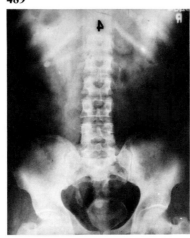

490

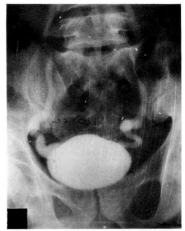

491

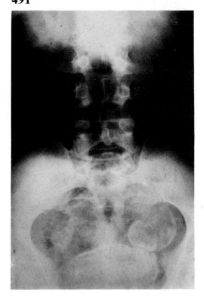

Bilharziasis of the ureter

In bilharziasis of the ureter the initial and subsequent pathology is the same as in the bladder. The commonest regions to be affected are the intramural part which is usually involved secondary to bladder pathology, then the juxtavesical part. Bilharzial changes in the ureter are almost always bilateral, although one ureter may be affected more than the other. The final result of the bilharzial infiltration of the ureter is dense fibrosis involving all or most of its layers; calcification is common.

489 **Plain xray showing contracted and calcified bladder** with calcified right ureter and stone in the right kidney. In mild fibrosis, diminution of tone will cause the ureter to dilate in front of the pressure head of urine, columar from the kidney, producing the typical spindle-shaped ureter of bilharziasis.

490 **Early intramural bilharzial infection of the ureters** leading to intramural, stricture and spindle-shaped dilatation of the ureter, especially of the left side.

491 **Plain xray of more advanced disease with calcification of the bladder** with bilateral spindle-shaped dilated and calcified ureters. When fibrosis proceeds further it brings about dilatation and tortuosity of the ureter, which assumes a small intestine-like appearance.

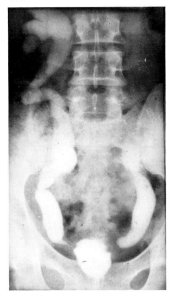

492

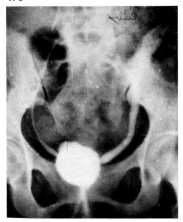

493

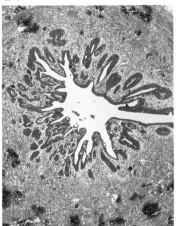

494

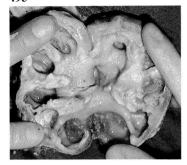

495

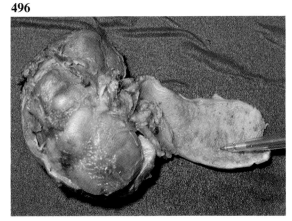

496

492 IVU showing: a) Severely contracted and irregular bladder; b) Severely constricted juxtavesical part of both ureters; c) Huge dilated elongated and tortuous intestine-like ureters with hydronephrosis. Contraction of the fibrous tissue produces also a stricture of the ureter at any level, usually in its lower third, but may be at the level of the third lumbar transverse process, with consequent proximal dilatation and tortuosity and with back pressure on the corresponding kidney.

Perivesical and periureteric fibrolipomatosis infiltration may press on the ureter from outside, adding to the ureteric obstruction and proximal dilatation.

Bilharzial ureteric reflux

493 Ascending cystogram with stage II ureteric reflux. About 96 per cent of bilharzial ureteric reflux cases result from bladder-neck fibrosis; infection is present in about 84 per cent of cases. Once reflux becomes established, progressive renal destruction usually follows, particularly in the presence of infection. Persistently severe bilateral reflux causes course scarring and back pressure atrophy of the kidney. Calcification is a secondary effect.

494 Ureter: schistosomiasis. A ureter with hyperplastic epithelium, a thickened wall and some calcified ova which are almost black and seen at the top and bottom of the field. *(H&E × 26)*

495 Infected hydronephrotic kidney with multiple big calculi in most of its pelvicalyceal system.

496 Infected hydronephrotic kidney, ureteritis cystica and calcinosis. Note the unhealthy, thick, dilated ureter with ureteritis cystica.

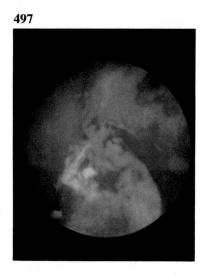

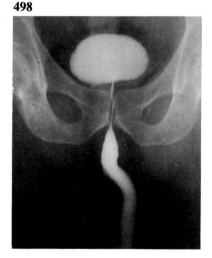

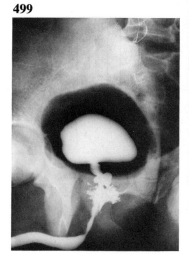

Bilharzia of the urethra

Urethral bilharziasis is usually associated with vesical and ureteral infection. The portal of entry of infection is through the deep dorsal vein of the penis from the pelvic pool of veins. The posterior urethral affection is a part of bladder-neck pathology giving congestion, hyperaemia, mild fibrosis and rarely ulcers.

497 Urethroscopic view of bilharziasis of posterior urethra with ulcerated bilharzial mass. The penile urethra is the commonest site of bilharziasis of the urethra. The ultimate result of bilharzial affection of the urethra is fistula formation, or stricture of urethra.

498 Bilharzial stricture of the posterior urethra. Note elevated bladder base secondary to bilharzial bladder-neck obstruction.

499 Urethral stricture with involvement of the prostate. Note again the raised and contracted bladder-neck.

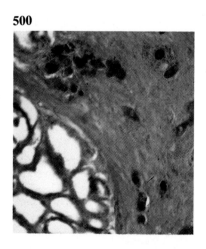

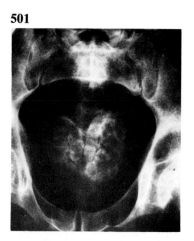

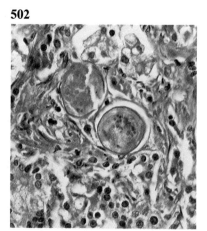

Bilharziasis of the seminal vesicles (SV)

500 Section of a bilharzial SV with multiple bilharzial ova. Note that the acini are not affected. The pathology starts in the fibromuscular part of the seminal vesicle and may remain as a closed lesion, or it may extend to the mucous membrane of the acini causing ulceration and secondary infection, ending in fibrosis.

501 Plain xray showing the honeycomb appearance of calcified bilharzial SV.

Bilharziasis of the prostate

502 Bilharzial ova in the prostate. The disease commonly occurs on the vesical and urethral surface of the prostate, because they are not covered by the thick capsule. One may get bilharzial nodules in the para-prostatic plexus of the veins, these nodules may be mis-diagnosed as calculus, tubercules or malignant nodules. This section shows ova in a prostate with adeno-carcinoma. *(H&E × 256)*

6 Calculi in the urinary tract

The incidence of calculi in the urinary tract is quite variable. This results from geographical differences, ethnic variations, the standard of living, diet and employment. Many calculi are an incidental finding and some calculi are passed without the patient knowing about it. Between two to three per cent of people in the western world develop calculi; 70 per cent of calculi are composed of calcium oxalate, with or without phosphate.

503   The common causes of urinary calculi.

Presenting symptoms

Patients with renal calculi may present with an attack of ureteric colic, loin pain, haematuria or recurrent urinary tract infection usually caused by the bacillus proteus.

504   A typical urinalysis for a patient with renal calculi.

503

Non-metabolic
Urinary tract infection
Prolonged recumbancy
Concentrated urine a) hot climate
b) chronic diarrhoea
Medullary sponge kidney
Matrix stones secondary to prolonged and severe urinary tract infection
Metabolic
Hyperparathyroidism
Hypercalciuria, caused by factors other than hyperparathyroidism
Idiopathic hypercalciuria
Medullary sponge kidney
Renal tubular acidosis
Vitamin-D overdose or sensitivity
Sarcoidosis
Paget's disease of the bone
Myelomatosis
Osteoporosis secondary to corticosteroid administration
Hyperuricaemia or hyperuricuria
Cystinuria
Xanthuria
Hyperoxaluria silica

504

HOSPITAL ....

Surname ....
Forenames ....
D. of B./Age................................. Sex ....
Unit No. .... Ward/Dept. ....
Consultant ....

Specimen Urine................ Mid Stream
Clinical details Recurrent Urinary Tract Infection with Renal Calculi
Antibiotic therapy Nil
Dr's. Signature .... Date................
Deposits Organisms & Sensitivities
Test wanted

Lab. No.:

p.H.	6.5	
Glucose	Nil	
Protein	Nil	
Micro:		
Pus cells	50/HPF	
Red cells	10/HPF	
Epithelial cells	Nil	
Culture:		
Viable Count	Profuse growth of B. Proteus	
	10^6 organisms/ml	

Antibiotic	1	2	3
Penicillin	R		
Streptomycin	R		
Tetracycline	R		
Sulphonamide	R		
Ampicillin	R		
Trimethoprim	S		
Nalidixic acid	R		
Negram	R		
Nitrofurantoin	R		
Gentamicin	S		
Cephradine	S		
Clindamycin	R		
Fusidic acid	R		
Methicillin	R		

MICROBIOLOGY
Specimen :
Tests performed :
Date received :
Date reported :

Investigations

It is mandatory that all patients presenting with a calculus in the urinary tract should have a complete investigation.

505 Summary of investigations required for patients presenting with calculi. If there is a persistently high serum calcium, hyperparathyroidism due to parathyroid adenoma causing hypercalcaemia must be suspected. Hyperparathyroidism is an important but unusual cause of renal calculi, being present in two per cent of all primary cases of urinary calculi and in up to 10 per cent of recurrent cases.

Investigations to exclude hyperparathyroidism include: Skeletal survey; Serum alkaline phosphatase which is always raised if there is skeletal involvement; and the cortisone suppression test. 100 to 150mg of cortisone a day for 10 days will depress a hypercalcaemia caused by sarcoidosis, myelomatosis, Vitamin-D excess, milk-alkali syndrome, and renal tubular defects and Paget's disease of the bone, but not in hyperparathyroidism. This finding in hyperparathyroidism is approximately 75 per cent accurate.

Discriminant analysis

The discriminant analysis is a multivariate analysis of biochemical data obtained from the plasma which is used as a discriminating procedure. The discriminant functions used are: plasma, inorganic phosphate, alkaline phosphatase, chloride, bicarbonate, urea and ESR. This test is used to differentiate between the causes of hypercalciuria. A recent survey of 168 patients at University College Hospital, London, when it was used in conjunction with the hydrocortisone suppression test, showed that it was 99 per cent accurate in distinguishing between hypercalciuria of parathyroid origin and that caused by non-parathyroid malignant disease.

506 Result of discriminant analysis in 168 hypercalcaemic patients. The circles around each group represent the area in which 95 per cent of the patients in each group would belong to.

Renal function tests, if secondary hyperparathyroidism is suspected; Urinary excretion of hydroxyprotein, which is used in cases of skeletal changes caused by hyperparathyroidism; Sampling of the venous drainage for estimation of parathormone by radioimmune assay.

506a Parathyroid adenomas may be single or multiple. They are difficult to diagnose and locate, but because the parathyroid hormone can be an estimated sampling of the venous drainage from different areas of the thyroid gland, intravenous catheterisation can enable a measure of localisation to be achieved.

Parathyroid tumour, either single or multiple parathyroid hyperplasia or rarely parathyroid calciuria, produce an excess of parathormone which causes disturbance of the calcium metabolism. In such instances calcium is increased both in the urine and the serum, and phosphorus is decreased in the serum but increased in the urine.

505

1 Intravenous urogram

2 a) Complete urinanalysis recording the pH and type of any crystals identified and any abnormal cystine content
   b) A proteus infection is commonly found in cases of recurrent stone

3 Chemical analysis of any stone passed

4 Serum urea electrolytes and liver-function tests

5 The measurement on three consecutive days of the fasting serum calcium, taken without venous stasis, inorganic phosphorus, plasma proteins with the A/G ratio, and uric acid, which is high in 30 per cent of cases of hyperparathyroidism

6 24-hour urine samples from which the 24-hour excretion of calcium, urate and oxalates are carried out

7 Radioisotope studies of the thyroid gland

8 Micturating cystourethrogram

9 Analysis of the stone

10 If cystinuria screening test is positive confirmation by electrophoresis for aminoaciduria

506

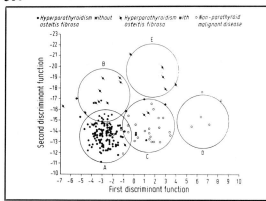

506a

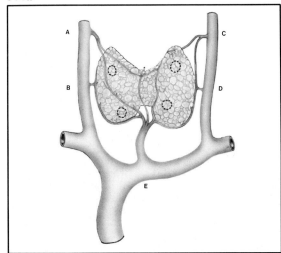

The high-serum calcium occurs as a result of the mobilisation of calcium from the bone because of the increased activity of the osteoclasis. This osteoclasis causes changes in the bone which may be the sole manifestation of hyperparathyroidism, but may also be associated with renal calculi or calcification in other areas of the body. The first change that may occur is a diffuse osteoclasis which results in generalised osteoporosis.

507 Generalised osteoporosis produces lack of mineralisation in the bone; the basketwork appearance is shown in the femur.

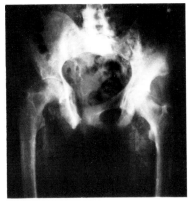

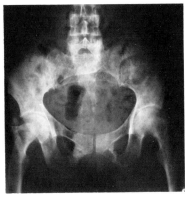

508 Pathological fracture resulting from demineralisation in the neck of the femur. Localised cystic areas may occur. They can be either multiple or single.

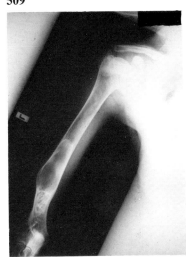

509 A cyst in the humerus. These cysts may have a thin sclerotic margin, but on the other hand they may show no evidence of dense surrounding bone. Fractures in this type of lesion are common. Localised subperiostial lesions are diagnostic of hyperparathyroidism. They are seen in the phalanges and are again caused by osteoclasis.

510   A subperiostial lesion. They may present as one or two small pits in the cortex of the phalanges of a finger or multiple pits which produce an irregular edge deep to the periostium. The latest stage is a lace-like pattern as seen; this is caused by the laying down of new subperiostial bone. Hyperparathyroidism can also cause calcification in other systems.

511   Diffuse calcification in the peripheral vessels.

512   Calcification in the pancreas combined with a staghorn calculus in a diabetic patient.

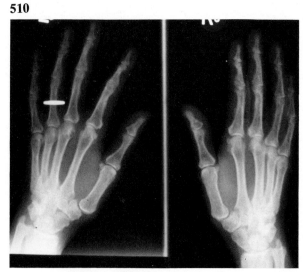

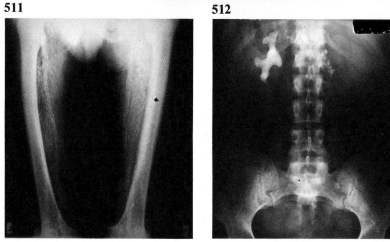

513

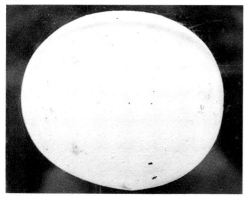

514

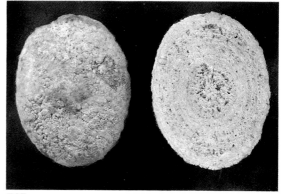

515

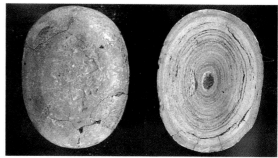

516

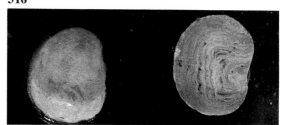

517

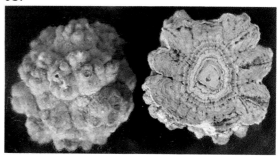

518

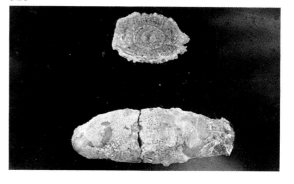

Composition of urinary calculi

A urinary calculus consists of a matrix of mucoprotein which is the core of the calculus. It is only a small part of the calculus contributing between 2.5 to 3 per cent of the total weight. The protein element is a mixture of a number of amino acids and the carbohydrate fraction is a combination of non-amino and amino sugars. In most calculi the matrix tends to be arranged in concentric laminations forming layers, as though it is essential for this arrangement to persist if mineralisation is to persist. The crystalline component is very variable and few stones are pure, i.e. consisting of a simple crystalline substance. The commonest is calcium phosphate with or without calcium oxalate and accounts for between 60 and 70 per cent of all urinary calculi. They are hard and can be smooth or irregular. One type is the mulberry stone, which is usually stained black due to blood pigment. 15 per cent of stones are composed of either spatite (basic calcium phosphate) or struvite (ammonium magnesium phosphate). These stones form in alkaline urine, are soft, rough and conform rapidly to the shape of the calyceal system. Metabolic calculi, most commonly of uric acid and very rarely of cystine or xanthine, are found in from 2 to 3 per cent of all cases of urinary calculi.

Examples of stones

513 Phosphate stone. This is regular, spherical and almost white.

514 Phosphate stone. The surface is irregular, and pitted, yet on section the laminations are clearly shown with the central areas.

515 Uric acid stone. They show a brown discolouration caused by blood pigment. The stones are softer and the laminations and central nucleus are clearly seen.

516 Uric acid stone. Another view, showing a more irregular stone, in which the core is close to the periphery, probably caused by the splitting of the calculus.

517 and 518 Two examples of oxalate stone.

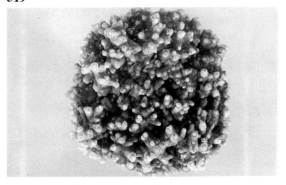

519   **Mulberry stone mostly oxalate.**

Amino acid stone

Cystine being most insoluble, there is a tree-like appearance with a very irregular surface and shape. The elongated shape is typical of a stone shaped to the pattern of a ureter.

520   **Cystine stone.** This stone is blue in colour, inter-spaced with white areas caused by a combination of amino acids. The finding of cystine on the urine screening must always be followed up by an examination of a 24-hour specimen for all amino acids by amino acid chromatography in affected patients; the worst cases are in the homozygous group.

Further examples of calculi

521   **Staghorn calculus (usually phosphate).**

522   **A mulberry calculus** removed from the kidney.

523   **An irregular-shaped calculus** removed from the ureter.

524   **Early staghorn calculus** with early branching.

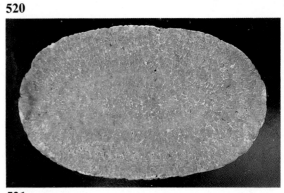

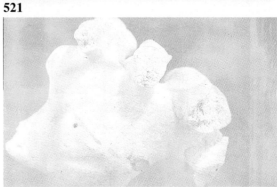

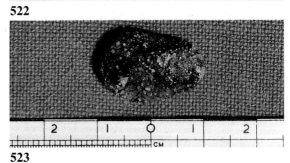

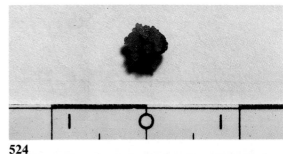

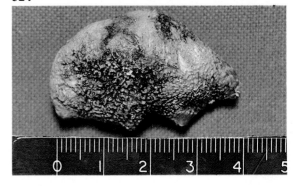

525

526

527

528

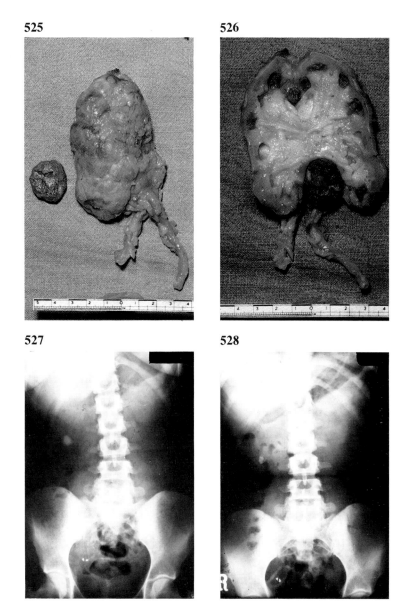

525 and 526 Two examples of the damage untreated calculi can cause. This calculus obstructed the pelviureteric junction completely destroying the kidney, which is shrunken, scarred with gross cortical destruction and with calculi in dilated calyces.

527 and 528 Two examples of cystine calculi. These stones are less dense, one showing the ring shadow, which is often seen. These calculi are from the same patient.

529

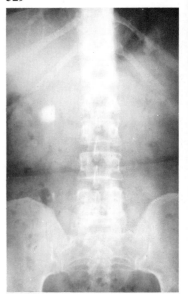

529 Example of a single calculus in the renal pelvis.

530 and 531 Straight *KUB and IVU of a small ring calculus in a calyx.

532 and 533 Straight KUB and IVU of multiple calculi in the dilated middle calyx.

*KUB is a plain straight abdominal xray film showing kidneys, ureters, and bladder.

530   **531**

532   **533**

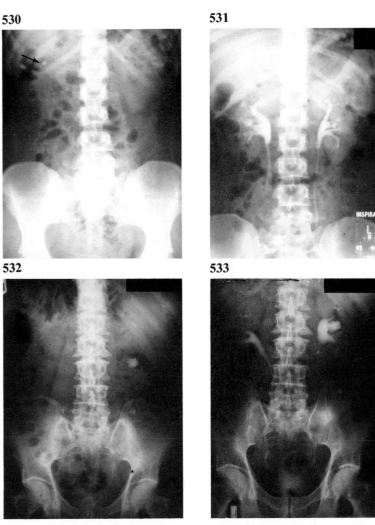

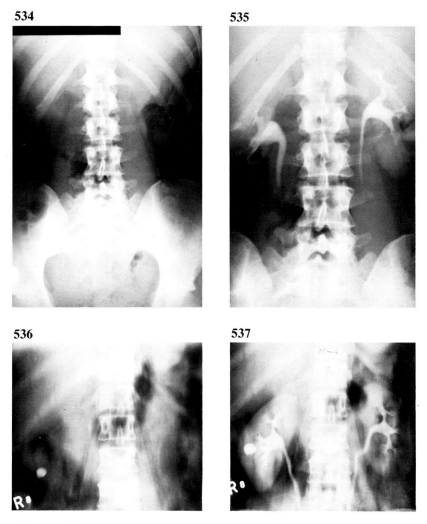

534 and 535   Straight KUB and IVU of a calyceal calculus producing cortical scarring.

536 and 537   Straight KUB and IVU showing large calyceal calculus producing minimal renal damage. This is a stone within a calyceal cyst.

538

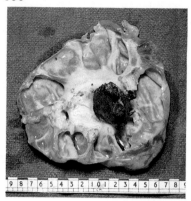

539

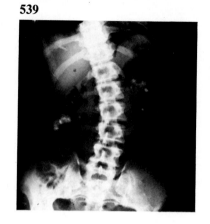

540

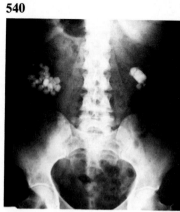

541

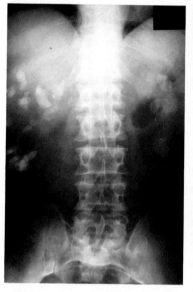

542

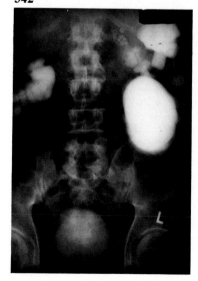

538 **Kidney destroyed by renal calculus**, which has obstructed the pelviureteric junction. There is almost total destruction, leaving only a thin shell of renal tissue.

539 **Multiple calculi**; note also the kyphoscoliosis.

540 **More extensive multiple calculi.**

541 **Very extensive multiple calculi.**

542 **Extensive calcification involving kidney and ureter.**

Uric acid calculi are not radio-opaque and are only diagnosed in the kidney when they produce a filling defect in the pelvis on an IVU.

543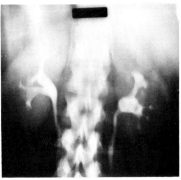

544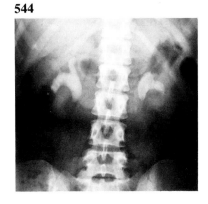

545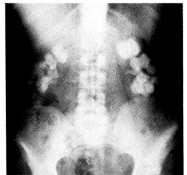

546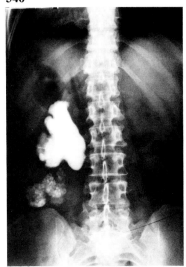

547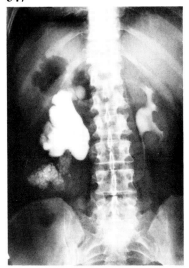

543   IVU of a filling defect in the pelvis of a kidney caused by a uric acid calculus.

Calculi can also conform to the pelvicalyceal system causing the classic staghorn calculus.

544   Early staghorn calculus which is beginning to branch.

545   Bilateral staghorn.

546 and 547   KUB and IVU of a staghorn calculus with an additional group of calculi in dilated lower-pole calyx.

548

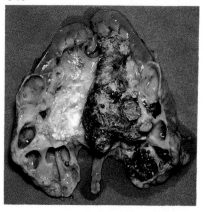

549

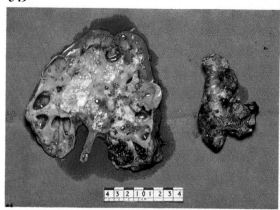

548 and 549 The effect of a staghorn calculus on the kidney, emphasising the seriousness of any neglected calculus.

550 Typical staghorn calculus pigmented. It was composed of calcium phosphate and magnesium ammonium phosphate.

551 and 552 IVU and micturating cystogram showing staghorn calculus which is secondary to ureteric reflux. This investigation must always be carried out in patients with staghorn calculi.

550

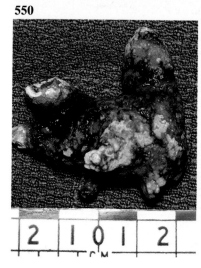

551

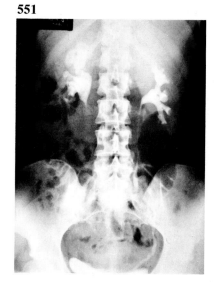

552

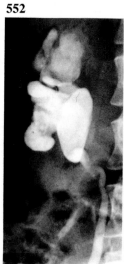

553

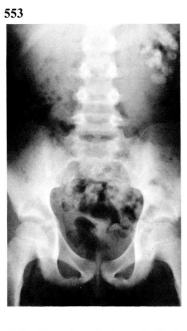

554

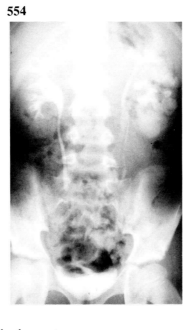

555

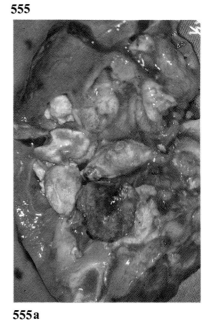

555a

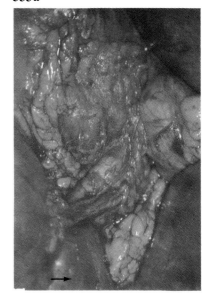

Calculi rarely affect one half of a duplex system

553   KUB showing multiple calculi in a lower moiety of a duplex kidney.

554   IVU of the same patient in 553.

555 and 555a Resected lower moiety containing numerous calculi.

Calculi may also be seen in a horseshoe kidney

556 and 557   KUB and IVU of a horseshoe kidney containing a single calculus in the left renal pelvis.

556

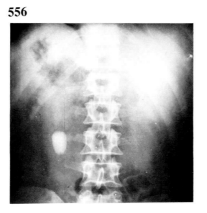

557

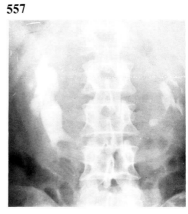

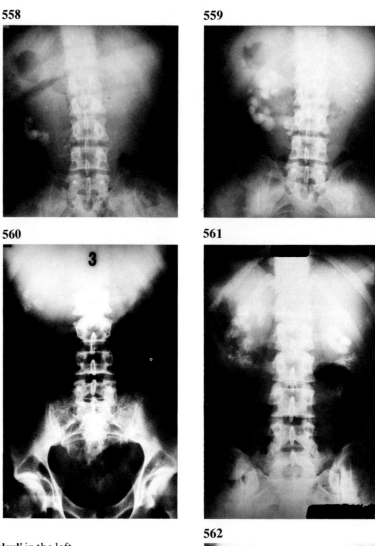

558 and 559   KUB and IVU of multiple calculi in the left pelvis of a horseshoe kidney causing pelvicalyceal obstruction.

Occasionally the calcium is deposited in the substance of the kidney and is referred to as nephrocalcinosis and this can be macroscopic or microscopic. The principal causes are hyperparathyroidism, malignancy, myelomatosis, Paget's disease of bone, renal tubular acidosis, medullary sponge kidney, Vitamin-D intoxication, the milk-alkali syndrome, sarcoidosis and idiopathic hypercalciuria. It may or may not be accompanied by renal calculi.

560   An example of early nephrocalcinosis.

561 and 562   KUB and IVU of severe nephrocalcinosis.

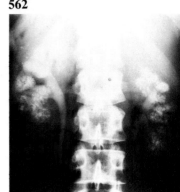

563 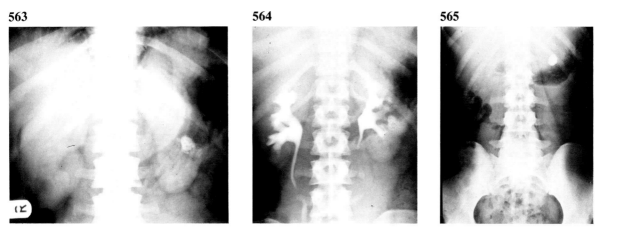 **564** **565**

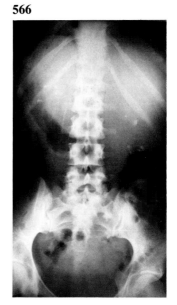

566

563 and 564 KUB and IVU of nephrocalcinosis accompanied by renal calculi.

565 An example of nephrocalcinosis accompanied by renal calculi. This patient also had hyperparathyroidism.

Calcification can also be seen in renal papillary necrosis. This is a late development and is due to calcification of necrotic papillae, which gives rise to a picture very similar to nephrocalcinosis. The commonest causes are diabetes, analgesic abuse, prolonged infection and sickle cell disease.

566 and 567 KUB and IVU of an advanced degree of calcification in papillary necrosis secondary to diabetes.

567

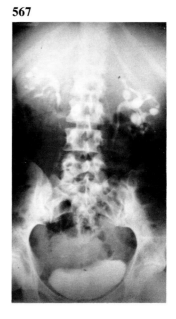

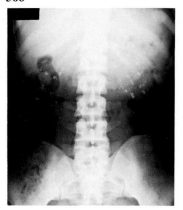
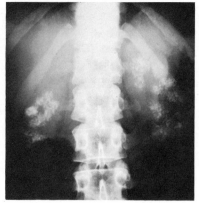
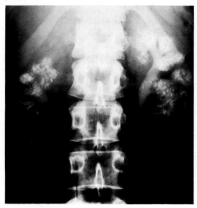

571

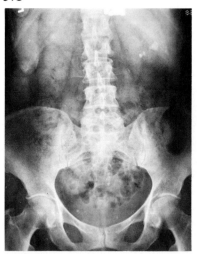

572

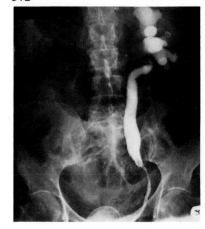

Renal tubular acidosis

Renal tubular acidosis is one of the causes of nephro-calcinosis. It is an inherited condition, transmitted by an autosomal recessive gene which leads to failure to acidify the urine. The characteristic presentation is a low-plasma bicarbonate accompanied by alkaline urine. The diagnosis is confirmed by the failure of the urine to become acid six hours after a loading dose of ammonium chloride, 0.1 gm/kg bodyweight over an hour. For this test to be accurate the urine must be sterile.

568 Case of renal tubular acidosis with calcification.
Medullary sponge kidney is usually recognised in middle age. It is manifested by small cysts in relation to the pyramids which on IVU appear as rounded cavities full of dye. They may be unilateral or bilateral and may or may not contain calculi. If calculi are present then the condition is difficult to distinguish from nephro-calcinosis. About 30 per cent of cases have idiopathic hypercalciuria. It is a congenital condition usually diagnosed after the age of 20.

569 and 570 An advanced case of medullary sponge kidney with calcification.

Ureteric calculi

Renal calculi may become dislodged and cause ureteric obstruction which produces ureteric colic; this will be the initial presenting symptom.

571 and 572 KUB and retrograde pyelogram in which part of a renal calculus has obstructed the ureter causing hydroureter and hydronephrosis.
Ureteric calculi can obstruct in the upper middle or lower third.

573

574

575

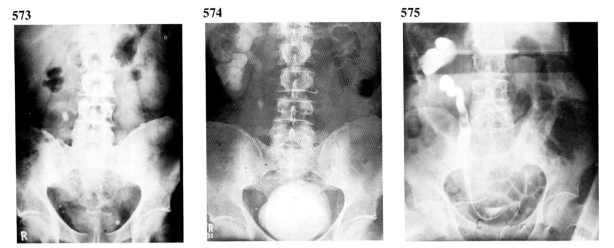

573   Calculus lodged in the upper third of the ureter.

574   Calculus lodged in the mid third of the ureter.

575   **Urate calculus which is almost non-opaque** to xrays obstructing the mid third of the ureter.

575 a

575 b

575a   **Ureteric stone.** A postmortem specimen of a ureter showing a bulge caused by a stone (in the centre of the field), a normal ureter below the bulge and a dilated ureter above it.

575b   **Ureteric stone.** The previous specimen dissected to show a unilateral hydroureter caused by a stone a short distance above the bladder.

576

577

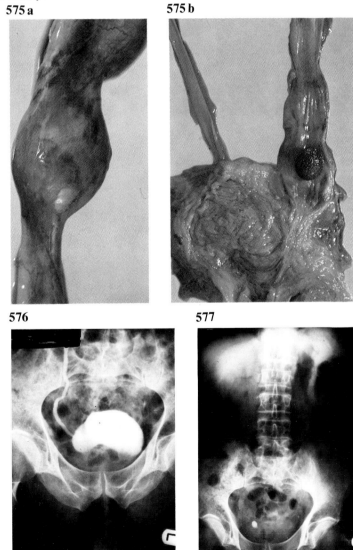

576 and 577   KUB and IVU of calculus situated in the lower third of the ureter close to the interovesical junction.

145

578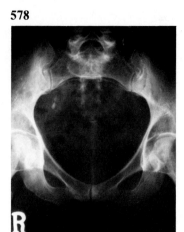

579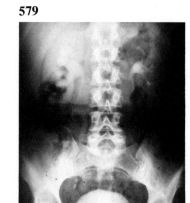

580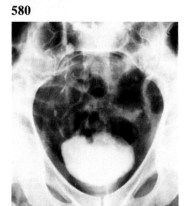

The effect of a calculus is unpredictable. Sometimes the same size of calculus causes obstruction as is shown in **578** and **579**. On other occasions there is free ureteric drainage, as **580** and **581** demonstrate.

581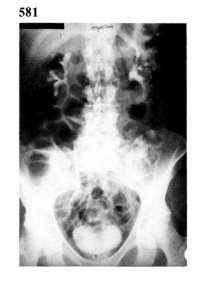

Ureteric calculi occasionally form in ureteroceles.

582 and 583 Calculus in a ureterocele which is at the lower end of the a duplex system. The ureters join just above the ureterovesical junction.

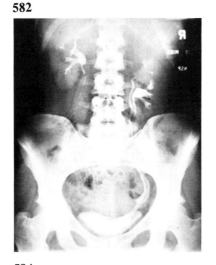

582

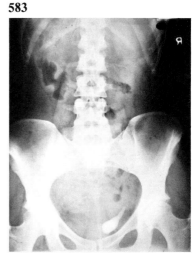

583

584 Multiple calculi in a ureterocele, kidney and ureter.
Large ureteric calculi can pass through the intramural part of the ureter.

585 A large ureteric calculus which passed spontaneously, though they require careful supervision.
Calculi of this size must be watched carefully, because they rarely pass spontaneously.

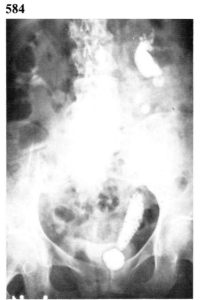

584

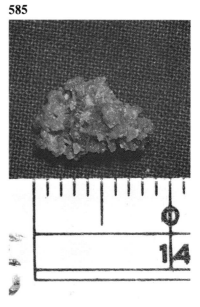

585

586 and 587 A calculus removed by a Dormia basket, a technique that can be used if the calculus is small and no ureteric dilatation is evident.

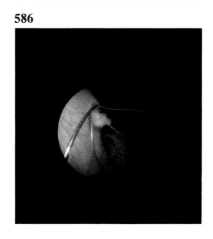

586

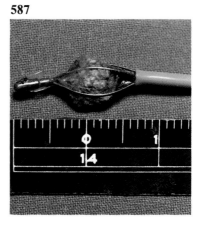

587

588 Dangers of using a Dormia basket. Breaking of the basket wire which becomes detached.

588

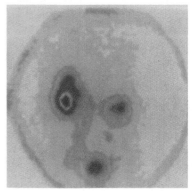

589

589 and 590 Radioisotopes in the investigation of ureteric calculi. Appearances 20 and 30 minutes after injection of I^{123} sodium iodohippurate.

IVU, the basic investigation of any renal symptom, can be of immense assistance in diagnosing early acute obstruction.

590

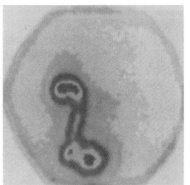

591

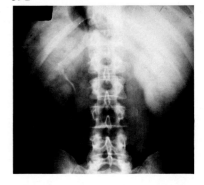

591 A dense nephrogram; a classical appearance in an acutely obstructed kidney. But this investigation has its hazards in the obstructed system.

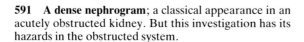

592 IVU showing spontaneous rupture in an acutely obstructed upper urinary tract.

Ureteric obstruction rarely seen today. Is due to sulphon-amide crystal formation.

593 Ureter obstructed by sulphamethizole crystals. Note the linear pattern and the filling defect in the bladder which is caused by blood clot.

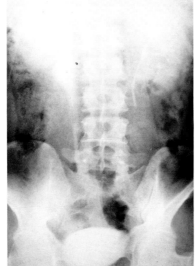

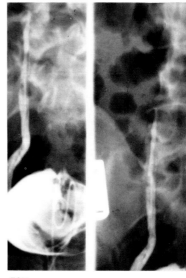

594 KUB of calculi present in the kidney, ureter and a bladder diverticulum. On rare occasions calculi can involve multiple parts of the renal tract.

Bladder calculi

Bladder calculi may be primary or secondary. Primary calculi are rare in the western world but are common in India, Pakistan, Iran, Egypt, and other middle eastern countries. Secondary calculi may be formed around a stone which has come from the kidney but are much more likely to result from bladder outlet obstruction. Calculi may rarely form over a foreign body which acts as a nucleus. They vary in size, colour, shape and number and their composition is similar to renal stones. Small stones must be distinguished from phleboliths, which are calcification in pelvic veins, are usually numerous and are situated outside the line of the ureter and lateral to the bladder outline.

595 Phleboliths.

596 Small bladder stone.

597 Larger bladder stone.

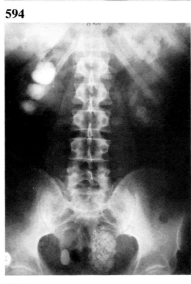

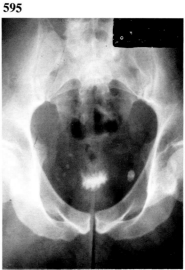

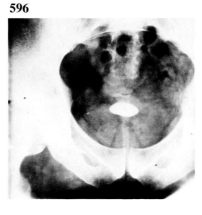

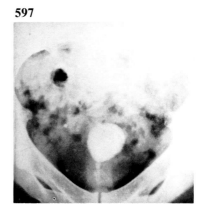

598

599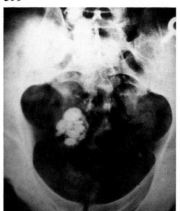

600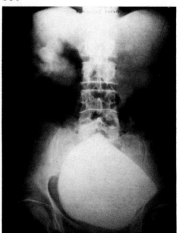

598   Multiple bladder stones.

599   Multiple bladder stones in a bladder diverticulum.

600, 601 and 602   Large bladder stone. This was
removed by one of us and weighed 2.1 kilos. The patient
ultimately died of squamous-cell carcinoma of the
bladder.

601

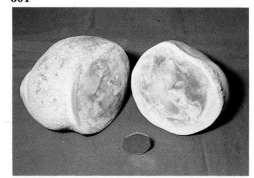

602

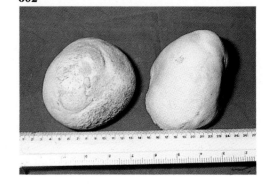

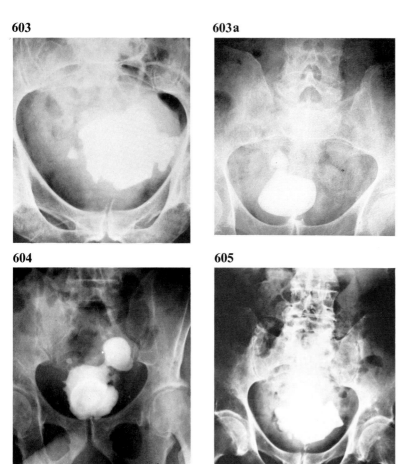

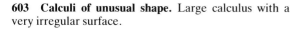

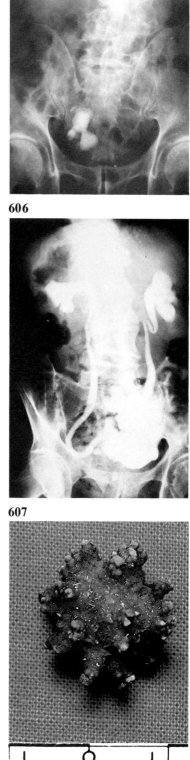

603 Calculi of unusual shape. Large calculus with a very irregular surface.

603a Single calculus in a diverticulum which has the appearance of a ring shadow.

603b Dumbell appearance.

604 Large calculus involving the bladder and a diverticulum.

605 and 606 Large calculus causing varying degrees of obstruction to the upper urinary tract.

607 Mulberry calculus removed from the bladder. It is identical to the renal mulberry stone.

608 Multiple mixed stones removed during a prostatectomy.

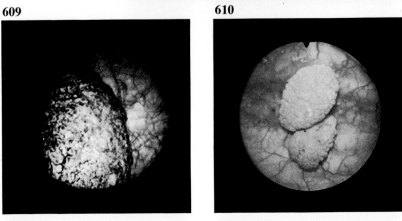

Endoscopic appearances of calculi

609 Mulberry stone with mild degree of cystitis.

610 Two irregular, rough calculi.

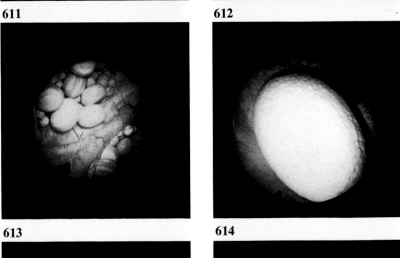

611 Outflow obstruction causing numerous small calculi. Note trabeculation.

612 A calculus with severe cystitis.

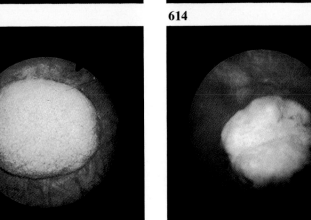

613 A calculus with a minor degree of inflammation.

614 A soft stone combined with severe infection.

615

616

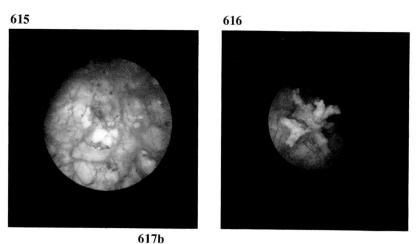

617a

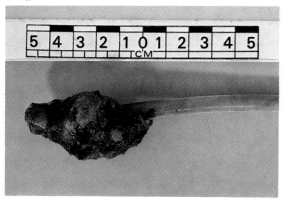

617b

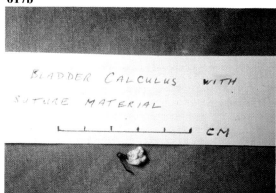

BLADDER CALCULUS WITH
SUTURE MATERIAL

CM

615 Multiple small calculi secondary to bladder outlet obstruction.

616 Endoscopic view of Jackstone in the bladder.

617a **Bladder stone.** A calculus forming on the tip of a catheter which had been left in the bladder for a long time.

617b **Calculi occasionally form over a foreign body.** Bladder calculus formed over non-absorbable suture material which had inadvertently included the bladder during pelvic surgery.

618 **Larger bladder calculus formed over suture material.** The calculus remained securely attached to the bladder wall. Part of the bladder had to be resected.

619 Calcification involves the whole of the thickness of the bladder wall.

618

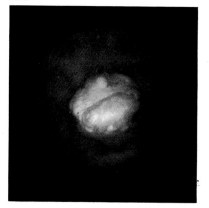

619

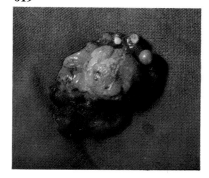

      621   622

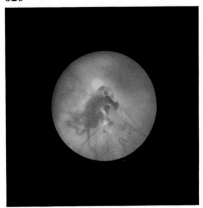 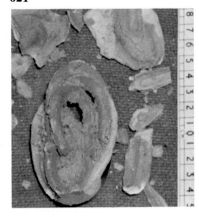 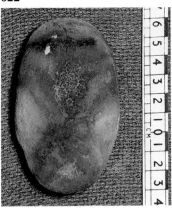

620 A rare cause of bladder calculi is secondary to irradiation cystitis. An area of irradiation cystitis on which small calculi have formed. They are usually pigmented and are basically composed of calcium oxalate.

Foreign bodies of many types have been reported in the bladder and most of these have been introduced along anatomical channels. Among many described are pieces of endoscopic instruments, a urethral catheter coated with phosphatic secretion, slippery elm bark, hair pins, safety pins, pencils, wire and paper clips. These are but a few of an almost endless number of bizarre articles.

621 Calcified catheter removed from the bladder.

622 Same foreign body before destruction.

623 Urogram of same foreign body.

Calcification occurs in the prostate and can be associated with bladder outlet obstruction. It is always multiple and may take the form of multiple prostatic calculi.

624 and 625 KUB and IVU of prostatic calcification associated with early bladder outlet obstruction.

623   624   625

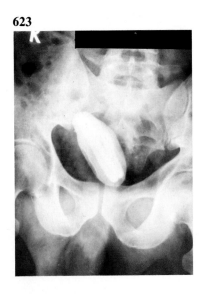 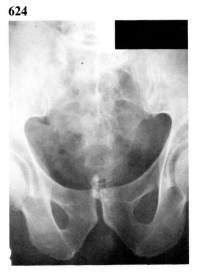 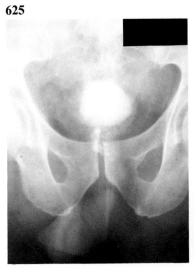

626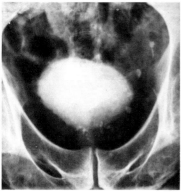

627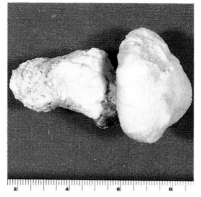

628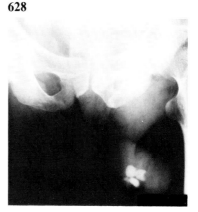

629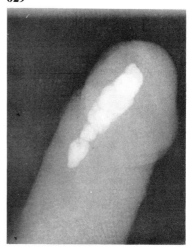

630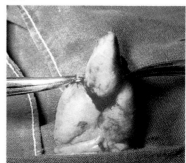

626 KUB of prostatic calcification associated with gross bladder outlet obstruction and trabeculation; note the numerous phleboliths.

627 Calculi removed from the prostate. Note the waist in the middle caused by part of the calculus being in the bladder and part in the prostatic urethra.

Urethral calculi

Calculi are occasionally found in the urethra. They are always secondary to bladder calculi unless they form in a urethral diverticulum and usually come to light when they cause urinary obstruction by being wedged in the urethra.

628 Calculi in a urethral diverticulum.

629 Spindle shaped calculus impacted in the penile urethra.

630 and 630a Calculus presenting at the urethral orifice and after extraction.

630a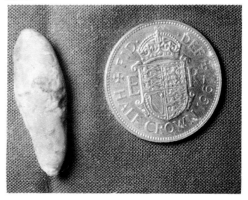

7 Tumours of the kidney and ureter

Patients with tumours of the renal substance, renal pelvis or ureter most commonly present with haematuria. They may also complain of loin pain. A loin mass may be present as a result of either the actual renal tumour, or as a result of hydronephrosis produced by ureteric obstruction.

Unusual presentations include haematological disturbances such as polycythaemia, pyrexia of unknown origin (PUO), and as a result of symptoms from metastatic deposits usually in the bones or in the chest.

Most of the tumours encountered in clinical practice are renal cortical carcinomas, nephroblastomas or transitional cell carcinomas. The other primary tumours are much less frequently seen. It is rare for a metastasis to present in the kidney but at autopsy secondary deposits in the kidney are not uncommon.

Tumours of the kidney

Renal cortical carcinoma	(Hypernephroma, renal adenocarcinoma, Grawitz tumour, renal carcinoma)
Nephroblastoma	(Wilms' tumour)
Connective tissue tumours	e.g. leiomyoma
Tumour like lesions	e.g. Hamartoma, solitary cyst.

Tumours of renal pelvis and ureter

Epithelial tumours	Carcinoma
Connective tissue tumours	
Tumour like lesions	e.g. Fibroepithelial polyp, malakoplakia.

631 Schematic representation of tumours of the kidney, pelvis and ureter.

Calcification is found in some renal tumours.

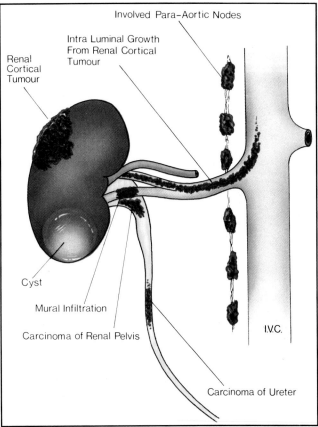

631

Renal Cortical Tumour

Intra Luminal Growth From Renal Cortical Tumour

Involved Para-Aortic Nodes

Cyst

Mural Infiltration

Carcinoma of Renal Pelvis

I.V.C.

Carcinoma of Ureter

632

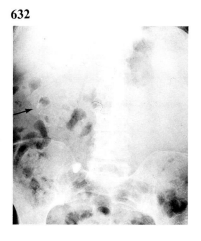

633

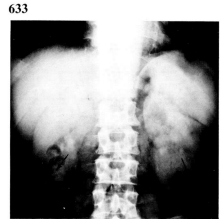

Plain xray of the abdomen

The renal outlines can be seen and here enlargement of the contour of the left lower pole indicates the presence of a space-occupying lesion, in this case a tumour.

632 Diffuse stippling in a right renal tumour.

633 Peripheral tumours may be defined with tomography.

Intravenous urography (IVU) is the most important single investigation in patients suspected of suffering from a renal tumour.

634 Calyceal distortion with stretching and separation of the calyces indicates a space-occupying lesion.

635 Calyceal destruction indicates tumour invasion of the drainage system.

636 The renal pelvis can also be invaded.

634

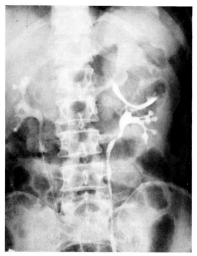

636

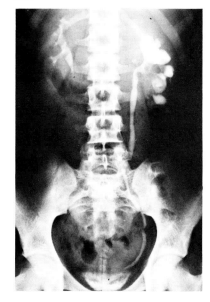

635

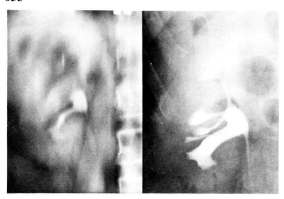

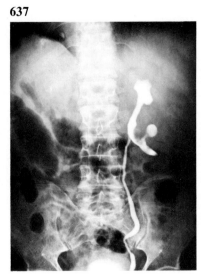

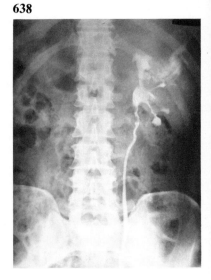

Ureterography

637 and 638 The technique of ascending contrast studies is invaluable in demonstrating destruction of the pelvicalyceal system in non-functioning kidneys.

Renal arteriography

This study demonstrates both kidneys by the flood technique or individual systems by selective arteriograms.

639 Flood films show the vascular pattern of both kidneys.

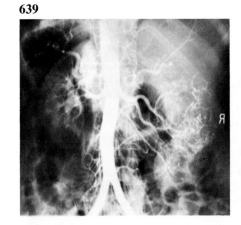

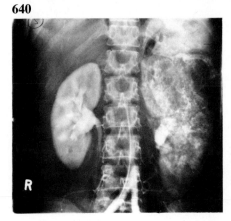

640 The late phase shows the normal right kidney with the enlarged left kidney showing diffuse tumour circulation.

641 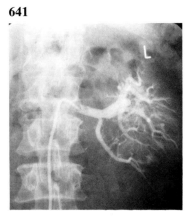 **642** 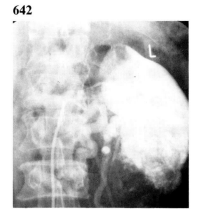 **643**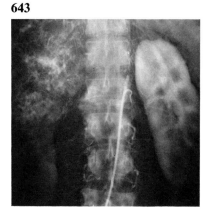

641 and 642   Early and late selective films demonstrate the vascular pattern in a renal tumour.

643   An example of the early phase shows the normal dense left nephrogram with the 'tumour blush' of fine pathological vessels on the contralateral side.

644   A selective film showing arteriovenous fistulae in a large tumour. Lakeing or pooling of contrast medium is present.

645 and 646   Subtraction films may be helpful. An IVU, arteriogram and subtraction arteriogram are shown here.

644 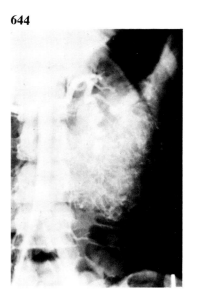 **645** 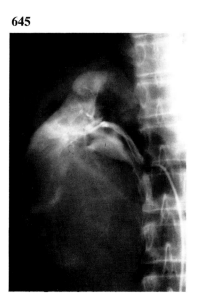 **646**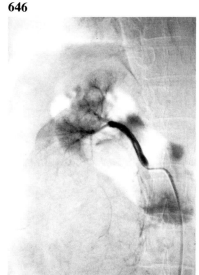

Vascular invasion

Spread of renal cortical tumours may occur, with extension of the tumour within the lumen of the renal vein and cava, and may invade the walls of these vessels.

647 **Dissection of the main renal vein** of a formalin fixed specimen with elevations on the inner wall of the vein, where the tumour in the kidney is growing through into the vein.

Cavography

648 **Tumour visible in the renal vein.**

649 and 650 **Early and late involvement of the cava.**

647

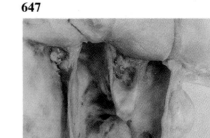

648

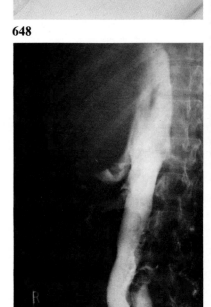

649

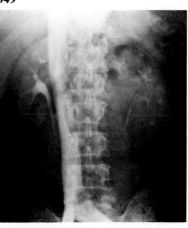

650

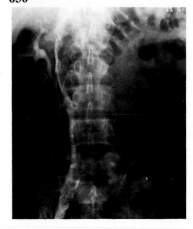

51a

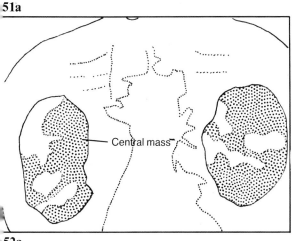

651b

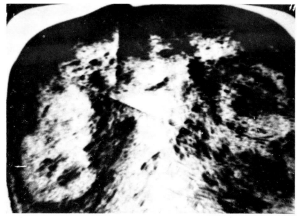

52a

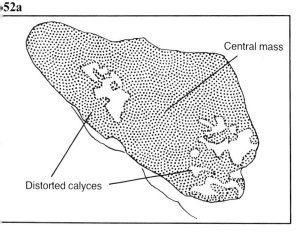

652b

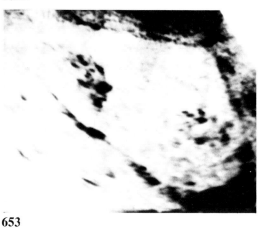

653

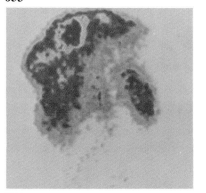

Ultrasound

This technique will show whether a space-occupying lesion is solid or cystic by the presence or absence of 'echoes'.

651a and b: 652a and b Transverse and longitudinal studies of a renal tumour (arrowed) demonstrating the echoes from the solid lesion.

Renal scan, posterior view

Left lower pole renal carcinoma

653 Vascular study. The picture is taken 15 to 30 seconds after a rapid injection of 99^{m}Tc-gluconate showing normal perfusion of the right kidney, but there is a prominent area of abnormal vascularity at the lower pole of the left kidney.

654 Parenchymal study. This gamma camera picture is taken 4 minutes later and shows normal uptake of the trace indicating normal function in the right kidney and the upper pole of the left kidney. No uptake, however, is seen in the lower pole of the left kidney.

654

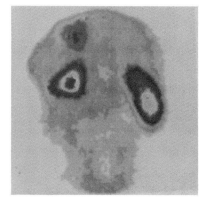

655

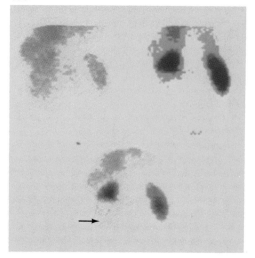

656

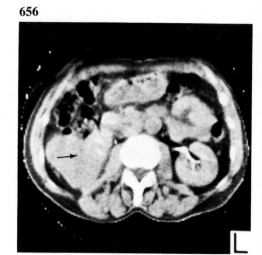

655 Supraimposing of vascular and parenchymal studies. The vascular study is shown in red, the parenchymal in green and confirm that the space-occupying lesion of the lower pole of the left kidney is vascular.

CAT scan

Computerised axial tomography of the renal image shows, on transverse abdominal 'cuts', the variation of density exhibited by the renal tumour and will also indicate gland masses when present.

656   A right renal tumour appears as a solid renal mass.

Chest xray

657   Classical appearance of 'cannon ball' metastases seen throughout both lung fields.

657

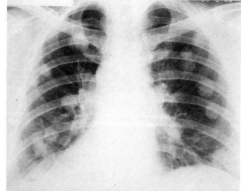

Bone metastases

658   Metastasis in the bone.

659   Pathological fracture in a weight bearing bone.

658

659

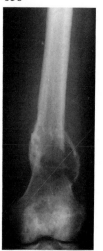
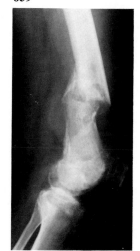

660

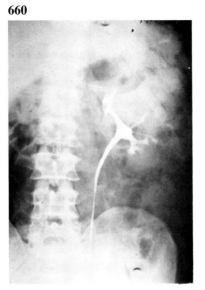

661

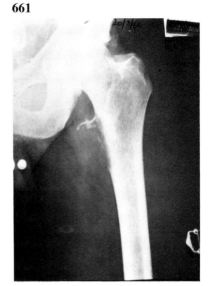

662

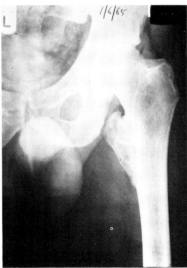

'Spontaneous regression'

A well-recognised but rare phenomenon occurs with the metastases from renal cortical tumours. After removal of the primary, pulmonary metastases can regress completely and bony metastases can recalcify without further treatment.

660   IVU of a renal carcinoma. 661 Note the osteolytic metastasis in the left lesser trochanter of this patient.

662   Recalcification of the lesion after nephrectomy, with no local treatment of the metastasis. The patient remains well and disease-free 17 years after surgery.

Typical renal tumours

663   Renal cortical carcinoma. A large tumour distorting the pelvis and destroying much of the middle of the kidney. It is apparently encapsulated and fibrous bands separate lobulated tumour masses.

663

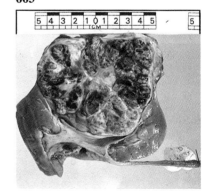

664

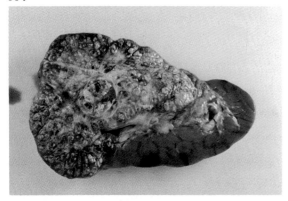

665

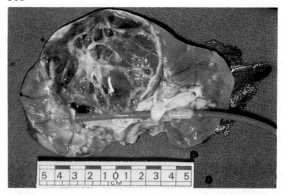

666

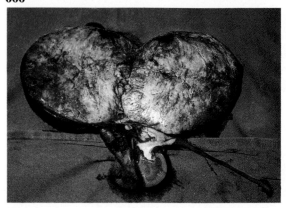

664 Renal cortical carcinoma. The whole of the lower pole is occupied by the tumour mass which has invaded the pelvis and extended through the capsule of the kidney.

665 Renal cortical carcinoma. This apparently encapsulated cystic mass is actually a renal cortical carcinoma showing widespread cystic change.

666 An encapsulated cortical tumour: a further example.

Renal cortical carcinoma

Renal cortical carcinoma is very variable in its appearance, even within the same tumour. Many patterns of cell growth can be recognised but they are all variants of the same tumour, which arises from the tubular epithelial cell. The variable pattern makes this tumour particularly difficult to diagnose in a metastasis – a characteristic which has earned it the reputation of 'The great mimic'.

667 Clear-cell pattern. The tumour cells here look fairly regular and the cytoplasm of most of the cells is clear. There is some tubule formation. The clearness may be caused by intracellular lipid or glycogen. *(H&E × 256)*

667

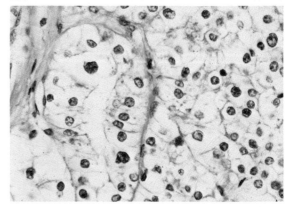

668

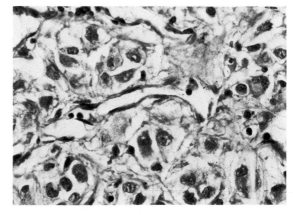

668 Granular cells. A small vessel in the centre is surrounded by tumour cells which have a rather granular cytoplasm. The granularity is a reflection of the many intracytoplasmic organelles in the cells of this pattern. *(H&E × 256)*

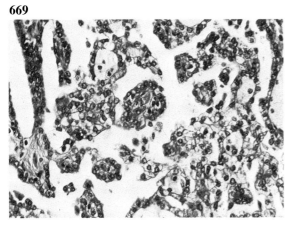

669

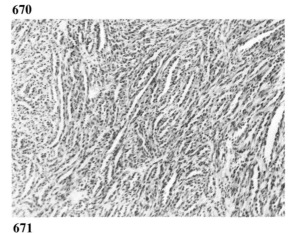

670

669 Papillary pattern. A tumour growing in a papillary pattern, i.e. the tumour cells are arranged as finger-like processes which have a core of connective tissue and vessels which is covered with the malignant cells. *(H&E × 160)*

670 Tubular pattern. Tumour cells are arranged in a well-marked tubular pattern. *(H&E × 64)*

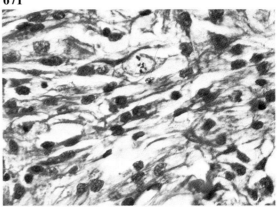

671

671 Spindle-cell pattern. Elongated tumour cells: they lie with their long axes parallel to each other. The appearances simulate those of a sarcoma rather than a carcinoma and may cause diagnostic difficulty (especially when the tumour presents as a metastatic deposit). Nevertheless, these cells can be shown to have epithelial characteristics. *(H&E × 256)*

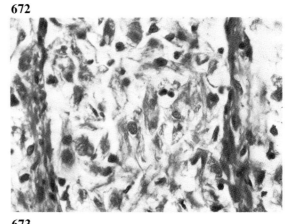

672

672 Vascular invasion. Tumour cells are seen in the lumen and surrounding a vein. This vascular invasion is a characteristic of renal cortical carcinoma and is associated with the high incidence of blood-borne metastases. *(H&E × 256)*

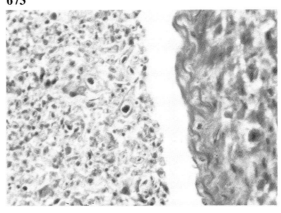

673

673 Vascular invasion. The arterial wall (on the right of the picture) abuts onto the tumour which has invaded into the lumen. The space between the wall and the tumour is an artifact caused by shrinkage during processing. Vascular invasion and occlusion of the blood supply to a part of the tumour may be responsible for the high frequency of necrotic areas within the tumour. *(H&E × 160)*

Aspiration biopsy

674 Cystic renal cortical carcinoma: cytology of needle aspirate. A clump of large cells in the middle of the field. The nuclei vary in size and the chromatin is irregularly clumped. The cytoplasm is plentiful, pale and slightly foamy. A renal cortical carcinoma was subsequently removed.

(The cells with small lobed nuclei are polymorphonuclear leucocytes.) *(H&E × 640)*

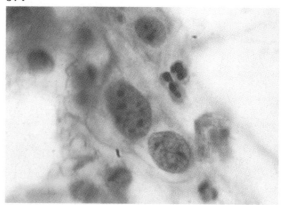

Adenomas

675 A scarred cystic kidney (acquired cystic disease following transplantation) in which there is a yellow nodule approximately 1.5cm in diameter in the cortex. Adenomas have an appearance similar to well-differentiated adenocarcinomas. They are unlikely to cause metastases if they are less than 2cm in diameter, provided that the histology is benign. They tend to be chance findings.

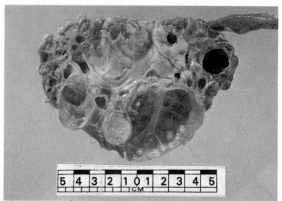

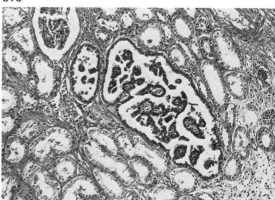

676 A microscopic adenoma. The normal tubules are seen around the periphery of the field. In the centre is a small adenoma, showing a papillary structure and composed of hyperchromatic cells. *(H&E × 64)*

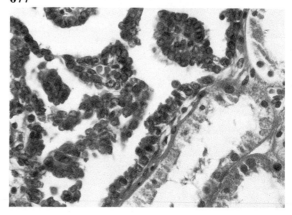

677 Papillary pattern. This picture contrasts the normal tubular epithelium (lower right hand corner) and the hyperchromatic cells arranged in a slightly papillary pattern in the adenoma. *(H&E × 160)*

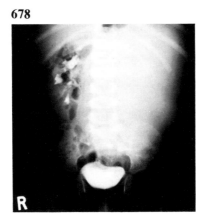

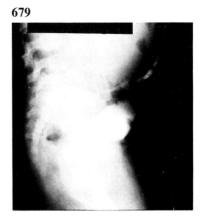

680

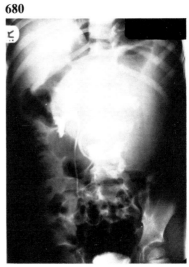

Nephroblastoma (Wilms' tumour)

This tumour is found exclusively in young children, and presents commonly with abdominal swelling and finding of the mass. One-third of the children present with haematuria.

Intravenous urography

678 Wilms' tumour. A mass can be seen to occupy the whole of the left loin.

679 Wilms' tumour. A lateral film shows dye in the pelvis stretched over the tumour mass.

680 Wilms' tumour. A smaller tumour causing calyceal distortion and displacement on the IVU.

681 Wilms' tumour. Multiple metastases may occur, very similar to those seen in patients with adult renal carcinomata.

681

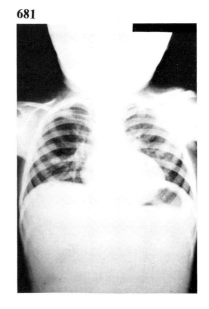

682

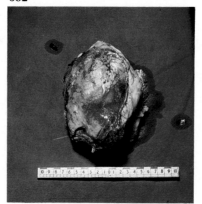

683

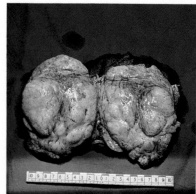

684

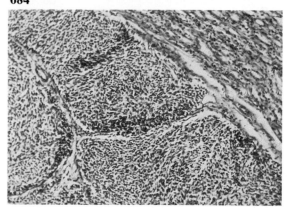

Examples of Wilms' tumour

682 and 683 Wilms' tumour. Whole of the kidney destroyed by this pale fleshy mass.

Microscopic appearances of Wilms' tumour

684 Tumour composed of sheets of small cells with dense nuclei and little cytoplasm. The normal renal parenchyma is seen at the top right hand corner of the picture. *(H&E × 64)*

685

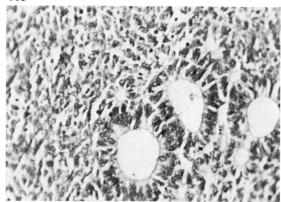

685 Higher magnification showing primitive tubules differentiating in a background of undifferentiated tumour. *(H&E × 160)*

686

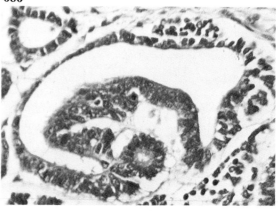

686 In some areas of the tumour structures resembling primitive glomeruli can occasionally be identified. *(H&E × 160)*

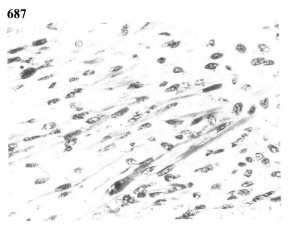

687 Area of tumour composed of elongated strap-like cells in which cross striations could be demonstrated. This is striated muscle differentiation in a nephroblastoma. *(H&E × 256)*

Leiomyosarcoma

688 **Leiomyosarcoma.** IVU showing abnormal calyceal pattern caused by a space-occupying lesion at the left lower pole.

689 **Leiomyosarcoma.** Arteriogram of the left kidney shows the classic appearance of microaneurysms similar to those seen in a hamartoma.

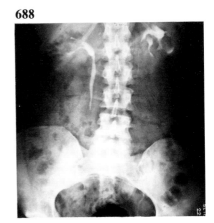

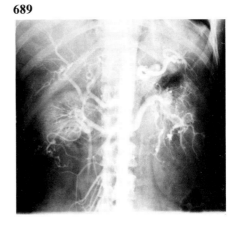

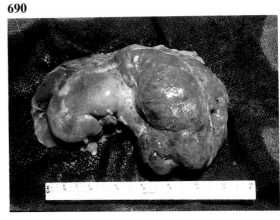

690 and 691 **An example of the rare leiomyosarcoma.** A brown fleshy tumour mass occupying one pole of the kidney and intruding through its capsule.

692 **Leiomyosarcoma.** Tumour composed of sheets or spindle cells with prominent mototic figures. Ultrastructurally the cells have smooth-muscle characteristics. *(H&E × 256)*

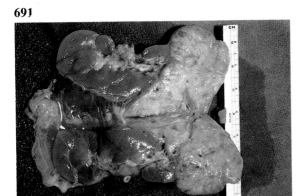

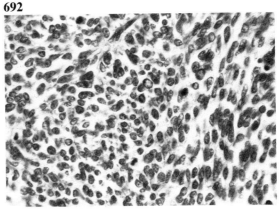

693

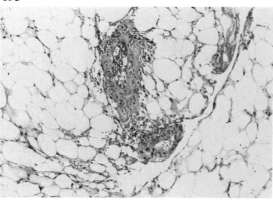

Angiomyolipoma

693 Angiomyolipoma is a hamartoma which contains tissue foreign to the part, and hence is properly designated a choristoma. It is primarily a non-neoplastic overgrowth of adipose tissue, thick-walled blood vessels and smooth muscle in varying proportions. Their developmental origin is shown by the fact that many patients with tuberose sclerosis have such lesions in the kidney, though they do occur in patients with no other manifestations of tuberose sclerosis. *(H&E × 64)*

694 Kidney: secondary carcinoma. This is a post-mortem specimen showing a large metastasis in the kidney of a man who died as a result of carcinoma of the bronchus.

695 Kidney lymphoma. This is a postmortem specimen showing multiple small deposits of tumour in a man who died from a disseminated non-Hodgkin's lymphoma (diffuse, stem-cell type).

694

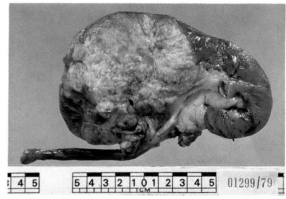

695

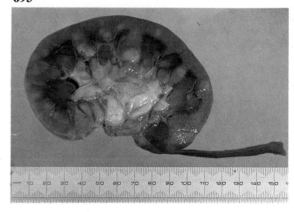

Cysts of the kidney (see also Chapter 2)

696a Cysts: IVU. The stretched calyceal distortion is indistinguishable from a solid space-occupying lesion.

696b Cysts: IVU. A space-occupying lesion in the upper pole.

696c Cysts: arteriography. An avascular area of the kidney with a well-demarcated edge.

Cystic disease of the kidney (solitary cysts)

696a

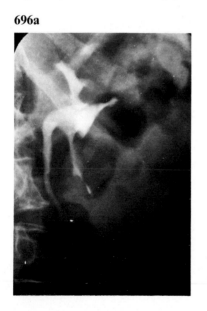

696b

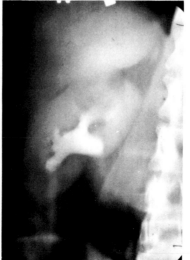

696c

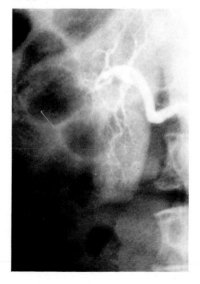

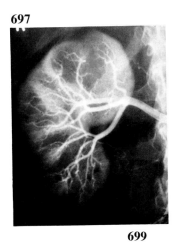

697

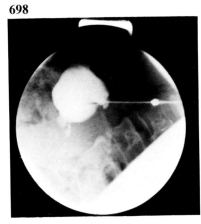

698

697 Cysts: arteriography. An avascular upper pole space-occupying lesion.

698 Cysts: puncture. Smooth internal surface of a cyst.

699 Cytology of this aspirate shows eosinophilic material in the background and a few isolated cells lacking any feature of malignancy. (Compare with **674**.)
(The cell with a lobed nucleus is a polymorphonuclear leucocyte.) *(H&E × 256)*

699

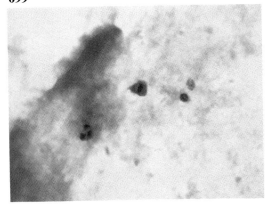

Ultrasound
700, 700a, 701 and 701a   Transverse and longitudinal views of a space-occupying lesion with complete absence of echoes.

700

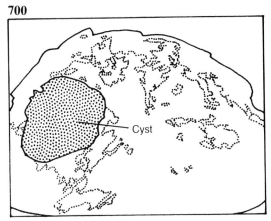

700 a

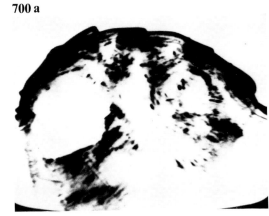

701

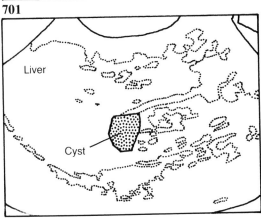

701a

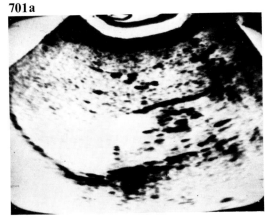

171

CAT scan

702 CAT scan demonstrates a well-demarcated spherical mass with altered and even tissue density indicating a cystic swelling. (arrowed)

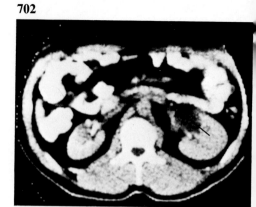

Cyst upper pole right kidney. Renal scan, posterior view

703 A vascular study showing a 'cold' area in the upper pole of the right kidney.

704

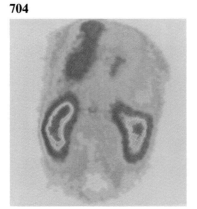

705

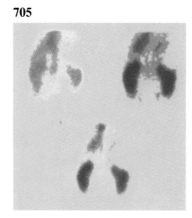

706

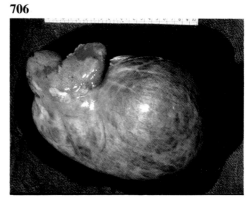

704 **A parenchymal study** matching the vascular study by showing a 'cold' area at the same time.

705 **Supraimposition of the vascular and parenchymal studies** shown in red and green respectively, confirming the presence of a non-vascular space-occupying lesion in the upper pole of the right kidney.

These should be compared with the scans of renal tumours, **653** to **655**.

706 **Macroscopic view of typical cyst** showing the classic blue-domed appearance.

707

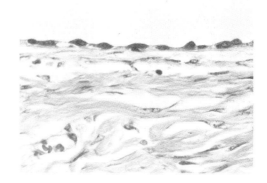

707 **Cyst lined by a layer of flattened epithelium** surrounded by fibrous tissue. *(H&E × 160)*

708

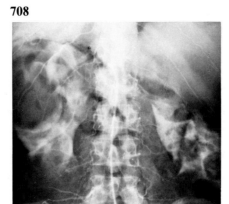

709

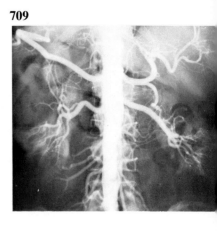

Intravenous urography

Tumours arising in the calyces or renal pelvis produce filling defects easily visible on urography.

708 Renal cystic disease encompasses many types of renal abnormality. Multiple cysts are found in one or both kidneys without progressive destruction of the kidneys towards end renal failure.

710

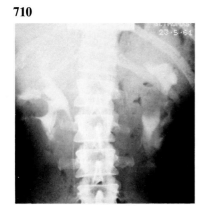

711

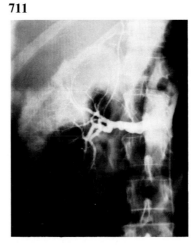

712

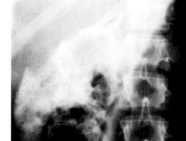

713

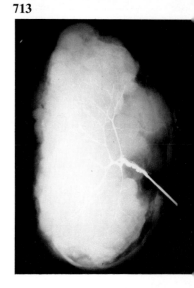

709 Arteriogram of patient with multicysts. Multicystic disease of the kidney is frequently symptomless, although haematuria and renal pain may occur. In contradistinction, polycystic disease of the adult kidney is a genetically determined condition which is bilateral and is slowly progressive, often leading to hypertension and end renal failure in adult life. Profuse haematuria may also occur, with loin pain when haemorrhage occurs into the cysts.

710 IVU showing bilateral enlarged kidneys with elongation of the calyces.

711 and 712 Arteriogram confirms the presence of multiple cysts.

713 Arteriogram of excised specimen.

This next series demonstrates the investigation of a solitary benign cyst of kidney.

714 Soft-tissue swelling of right kidney (arrowed).

715 IVU of a space-occupying lesion.

716 Selective renal arteriogram. Arterial phase outlines avascular cyst.

717 Venous phase of arteriogram: normal renal tissue surrounding cyst.

718 Ultrasound views confirm presence of cystic lesion (arrowed).

719 Cyst puncture: smooth internal surface of a benign cyst.

714

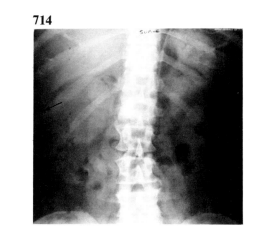

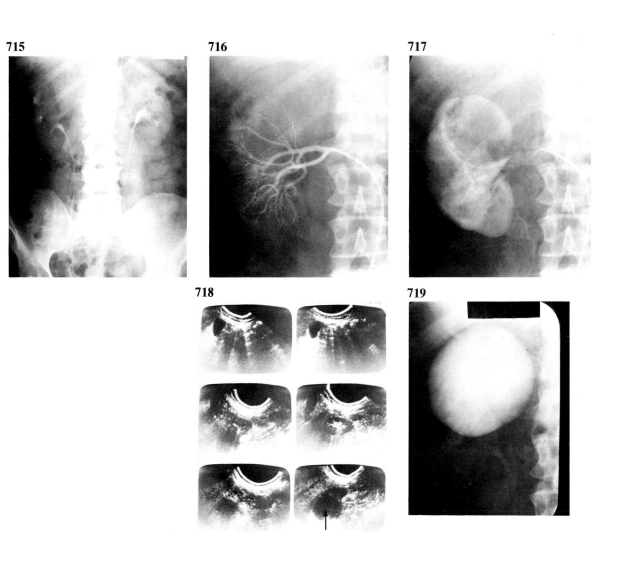

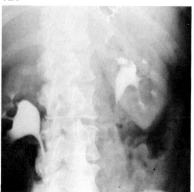

720

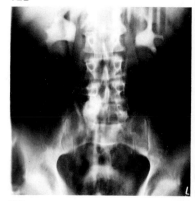

721

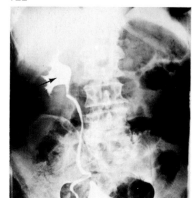

722

Tumours of renal pelvis and ureter

720 Tumour related to left upper calyx.

721 Tumour in right renal pelvis.

Ascending ureterography is invaluable for defining pelvic filling defects.

722 Filling phase. Lesion almost obscured (arrowed).

723 Emptying phase. Tumour well defined (macroscopic specimen **727**).

Arteriographic studies are usually normal, but occasionally pathological vessels can be seen in the region of the renal pelvis.

724 Arteriogram showing abnormal vascular pattern.

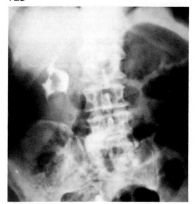

723

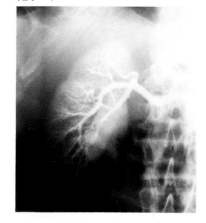

724

Urine cytology is often positive because these tumours are in the main transitional-cell carcinomata.

725 Cytological examination of the urine is useful in detecting carcinoma of the renal pelvis and ureter. This specimen showed many clumps of cells like those in the centre of the field. They are transitional cells with some atypical features. The patient was shown to have a transitional cell carcinoma (see also **776** and **777**). *(H&E × 256)*

725

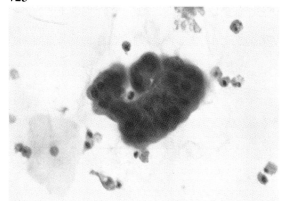

726

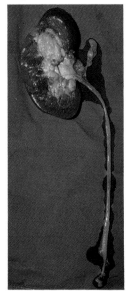

727

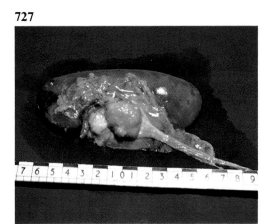

728

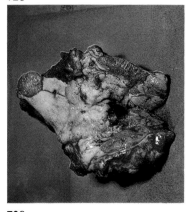

729

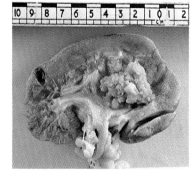

Transitional-cell carcinoma of pelvis

726 Tumour arising in the pelvis in relation to the upper calyx is a papillary differentiated transitional-cell carcinoma. No invasion was seen, but the renal parenchyma adjacent to the tumour showed fibrosis and chronic inflammatory changes.

727 Pelvis opened to show a rounded tumour sitting in the pelvis and growing into its lumen. This is a papillary, differentiated transitional-cell carcinoma.

728 Kidney opened to show a papillary tumour close to the pelviureteric junction. Proximal to this the pelvis is dilated and the kidney shows scarring. These effects are caused by tumour obstruction.

729 Papillary tumour. This specimen, which has been fixed in formalin and bisected, shows a papillary tumour involving the pelvis and calyceal system.

Ureteric tumours

Intravenous urography

Single or multiple tumours may appear as filling defects. Hydronephrosis and hydro-ureter may occur down to the level of the ureteric tumour.

730 Where complete ureteric stenosis occurs, non-function of that kidney will result.

Ascending ureterography

731 Ureteric tumours are well defined by retrograde studies.

Urine cytology

As with pelvic tumours, this is usually positive. (See **725**).

732 and 733 **Hydronephrotic kidney** caused by combined pelvic and ureteric tumours.

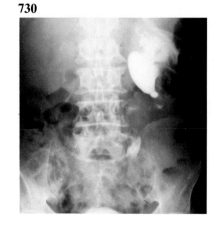

730

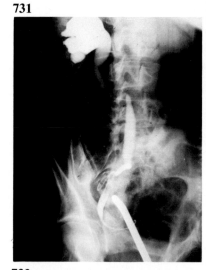

731

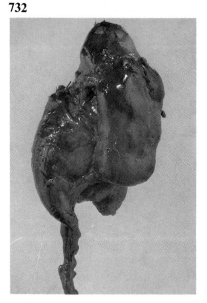

732

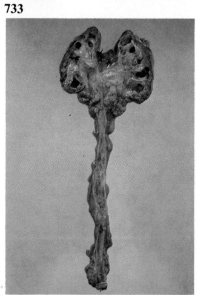

733

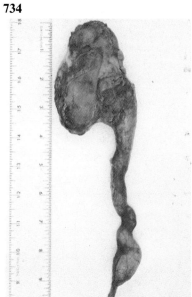

734

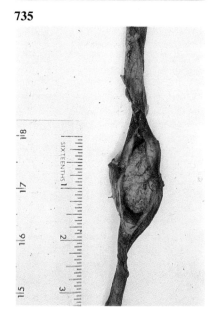

735

734 and 735 **Ureteric tumour** obstructing ureter and resulting in hydroureter and hydronephrosis.

178

736

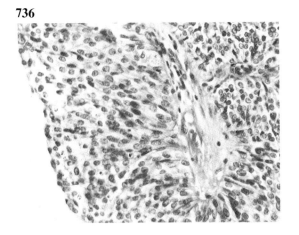

737

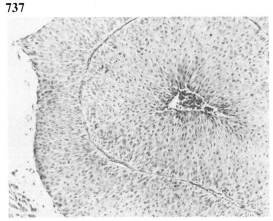

Transitional-cell carcinoma of renal pelvis

These tumours have a similar histological appearance to carcinomas arising further down the urethelial tract.

Transitional-cell carcinoma of ureter

736   A section of a papillary differentiated transitional-cell carcinoma. *(H&E × 160)*

737   Histology of 734 and 735. A papillary differentiated transitional-cell carcinoma.

738

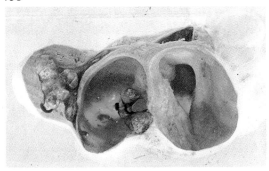

Squamous carcinoma of renal pelvis

738   The kidney has a bifid pelvis. The calyces of the upper pole are filled by a calculus. Another calculus is lodged at the pelvic bifurcation and the calyces arising from the lower portion are dilated; the corresponding renal tissue is atrophied. A warty tumour is seen arising from the lining of these calyces.

Histology showed a keratinising squamous carcinoma arising in squamous epithelium, associated with hydronephrosis and stones.

739

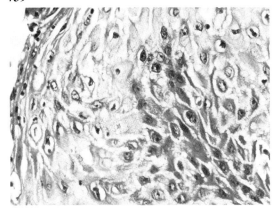

Kidney. Squamous metaplasia

739   Squamous epithelium lining a hydronephrotic pelvis. This is squamous metaplasia, i.e. the type of epithelium has changed from a transitional to a squamous type. There are also some atypical changes in these cells. These changes often arise in relation to the presence of calculi and infection. *(H&E × 256)*

740

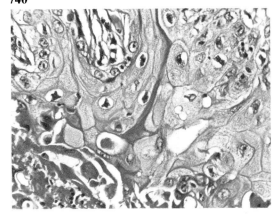

740   Sometimes carcinomas arising in the renal pelvis show squamous differentiation. This tumour shows large cells, resembling those of the prickle cell layer of the skin and keratin formation. *(H&E × 256)*

741 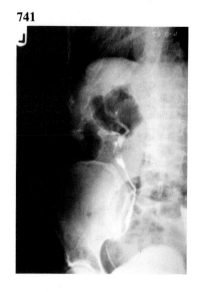 **742**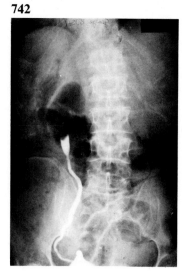

Ureteric polyp

741 IVU showing filling defect in ureter simulating carcinoma.

742 Ascending ureterography demonstrates the smooth meniscus effect, again difficult to differentiate from ureteric carcinoma.

743 The polyp consists of a core of connective tissue and vessels covered with transitional epithelium. *(H&E × 26)*

744 A higher magnification of 732 showing the bland appearance of the epithelium and of the fibrous core. There is no evidence of malignancy and the lesion is best called a fibroepithelial polyp. *(H&E × 160)*

743 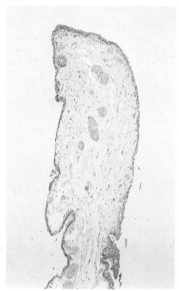 **744**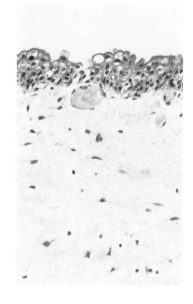

745

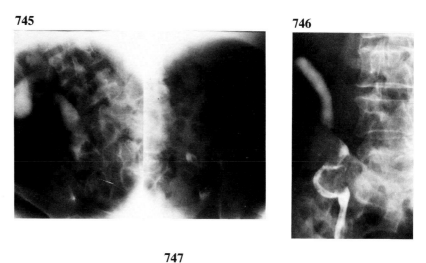

746

747

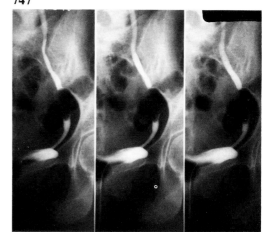

745   Bilateral ureteric tumour.

746 and 747   Tumour filling defect. Retrograde studies also well delineate the ureteric filling defect of the tumour.

748   A proliferative lower ureteric carcinoma.

749   Endometriosis may rarely involve the ureter, producing ureteric obstruction by stricture, as shown here in this ascending study.

748

749

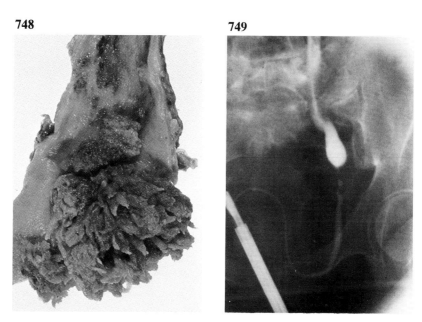

750

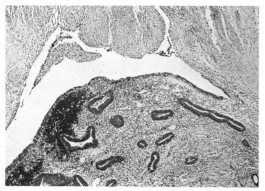

751

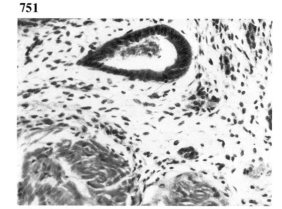

752

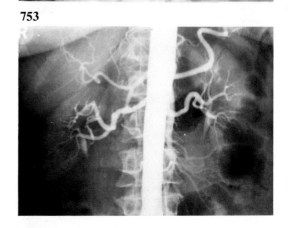

753

754

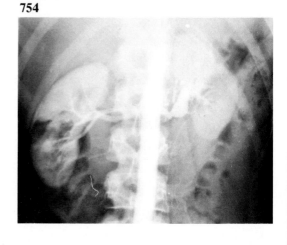

750 Ureteric endometriosis. In the lower part of the field there is a tumour-like mass composed of glands and stroma. This is endometriosis. These glands can be mis-diagnosed as adenocarcinoma by the unwary. Though they may show mitoses they lack other features of malignancy. The stroma is the clue.

751 Endometriosis. A higher magnification shows an endometrial gland with its loose stroma, the combination constituting endometriosis. The diagnosis cannot be made without identifying glands and stroma. At the bottom of the field ureteric smooth muscle is seen.

Renal artery stenosis

Hypertension may accompany many forms of renal disease and particularly when this is unilateral. Although uncommon, renal artery disease is well recognised as a cause of renal hypertension. Athero-matous plaques within the lumen, and fibromuscular disorders of the vessel itself are the mechanisms of this process. Renal size is frequently reduced on the side of the lesion.

The classical pyelographic findings are those of delay in excretion on the affected side with relatively increased concentration in later films caused by slow transit through the kidney. Divided renal function studies have now largely been replaced by renography and renal scans. Measurements of plasma renin or angiotensin are often used. Where the ratio of plasma renin activity from the stenosed versus the contralateral kidney exceeds 1.5, this is felt to be significant in most cases in assessment of the effects of the stenosis.

752 IVU of patient with hypertension reveals a smaller right kidney with increased concentration of the dye on that side.

753 Flood renal arteriogram: classic fibromuscular hyperplasia of the right renal artery.

754 Post-stenotic dilatation of this left renal artery caused by an atheromatous stricture.

755 Another leftsided stricture with an associated small kidney.

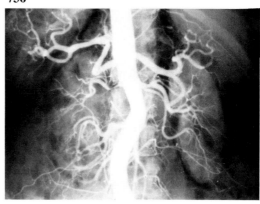

755

756 Bilateral arterial disease is present, and is more pronounced on the left.

756

757

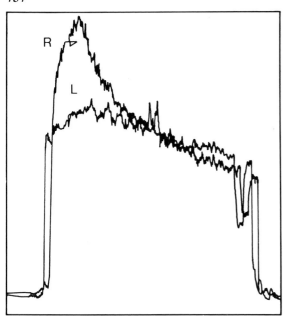

758

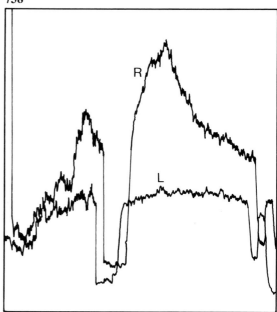

Renal artery stenosis

757 I^{131} Hippuran renography shows a normal right trace, but on the left the uptake and transit phases are both abnormal and reduced, due to the arterial stenosis on that side.

758 A further trace in a patient with a more marked and longstanding stenosis shows very little uptake or evidence of function on the left side. The right is again normal.

759 Renal artery stenosis. Nephrectomy specimen. This hemisection shows a small kidney with narrowed cortex associated with a renal artery stenosis. This kidney does not show gross scarring.

759
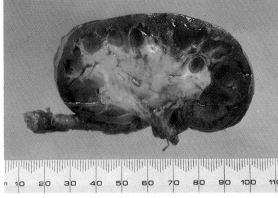

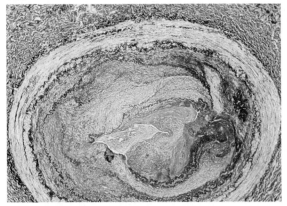

760 Renal artery stenosis. Section through a renal artery showing fibroelastic internal proliferation giving marked narrowing of the lumen. *(Elastic van Gieson)*

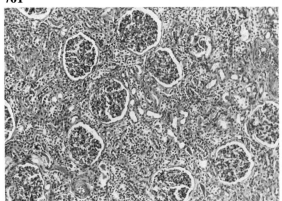

761 Renal artery stenosis. Section through the cortex showing glomeruli surviving among atrophic tubules. Glomeruli are crowded together because of the tubular atrophy. *(H&E × 64)*

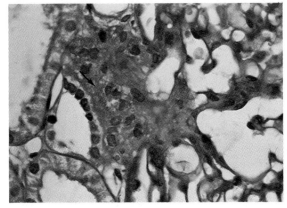

762 Renal artery stenosis. When glomerular ischaemia is present there is often hyperplasia of the juxta glomerular apparatus (arrow).

This group of cells is found at the hilum of the glomerulus. It is made up of cells of the afferent arterioles, the macula densa of the distal convoluted tubule and the cells of Goormaghtigh, which are continuous with the cells of the glomerular mesangium, which are on the right of the field. *(PAS × 400)*

8 Bladder tumours

The investigation and treatment of bladder tumours take up a major portion of a urologist's time. Although advances in therapy of this complex subject have been slow and unspectacular, a better recognition of the many aspects of the problem have allowed urologists to be more specific and precise in their approach to the different types of tumour. If this approach is to be progressive a pathological classification is essential.

763

I Epithelial	Benign	Transitional-cell papilloma Inverted type of transitional-cell papilloma Squamous papilloma
	Malignant	Transitional-cell carcinoma Squamous-cell carcinoma Adenocarcinoma Undifferentiated carcinoma
II Non-epithelial	Benign	Soft-tissue lesions e.g. leiomyoma
	Malignant	Rhabdomyosarcoma Others e.g. leiomyosarcoma
III Miscellaneous	e.g.	Phaeochromocytoma, lymphoma, carcinosarcoma, malignant melanoma

763 Classification of urinary bladder tumours.

About 95 per cent of bladder tumours are epithelial in origin and, in western countries, about 95 per cent of these are of transitional-cell type. Carcinomata are further characterised in terms of growth pattern (papillary or solid, or both), histological grading (degree of differentiation), staging (extent of spread) and type of spread.

764 Diagrammatic representation of the classification adapted from the UICC.
The UICC classification enables the clinician to describe and record bladder tumour data in internationally accepted terms. The extent or 'stage' of the primary tumour (T) with assessment of the presence or absence of local spread (T 1–4), lymphatic (N) and distant metastases (M) can thus be described. The pathologist will then examine any available tissue to determine the extent of spread of the disease or histopathological stage (P), and microscopy will demonstrate the histopathological grade or degree of differentiation of the primary tumour (G).

764

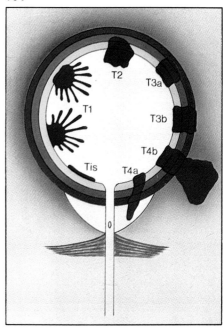

Table: Classification of tumours.

The meaning of the TNM symbols are as follows:

T   Clinical examination, urography, cystoscopy, bimanual examination under full anaesthesia and biopsy or transurethral resection of the tumour before definitive treatment.

N   Clinical examination, lymphography and urography.

M   Clinical examination, chest xray and biochemical tests and the more advanced primary tumours or when clinical suspicion warrants, radiographic isotope studies should be done.

Classification as applied to bladder tumours:

T   Primary tumour.

Tls   Pre-invasive carcinoma, carcinoma in situ. 'Flat tumour.'

Ta   Papillary non-invasive carcinoma.

Tx   The minimal requirements to assess fully the extent of the primary tumour cannot be met.

To   No evidence of primary tumour.

Tl   On bimanual examination a freely mobile mass may be felt. This should not be felt after complete transurethral resection of the lesion and/or microscopically the tumour does not extend beyond the lamina propria.

T2   On bimanual examination there is induration of the bladder wall which is mobile. There is a no residual induration after complete transurethral resection of the lesion and/or there is microscopic invasion of superficial muscle.

T3   On bimanual examination induration or a nodular mobile mass is palpable in the bladder wall, which persists after transurethral resection of the resection of the exophytic part of the lesion and/or there is microscopic invasion of deep muscle or of extension through the bladder wall.

T3a   Invasion of deep muscle.

T3b   Invasion through the bladder wall.

T4   Tumour fixed or invading neighbouring structures and/or there is microscopic evidence of such an involvement.

T4a   Tumour invading prostate, uterus or vagina.

T4b   Tumour fixed to the pelvic wall and/or infiltrating the abdominal wall.

N   *Regional and juxta-regional lymph nodes*

NO   No evidence of regional lymph node involvement.

N1   Evidence of involvement of a single homolateral regional lymph node.

N2   Evidence of involvement of contralateral or bilateral or multiple regional lymph nodes.

N3   Evidence of involvement of fixed regional lymph nodes (there is a fixed mass on the pelvic wall with a free space between this and the tumour).

N4   Evidence of involvement of juxta-regional lymph nodes.

NX   The minimum requirements to assess the regional and/or juxta-regional lymph nodes cannot be met.

M   *Distant metastases*

MO   No evidence of distant metastases.

M1   Evidence of distant metastases.

MX   The minimum requirements to assess the presence of distant metastases cannot be met.

Staging may also be carried out by the pathologist:

Histopathological categories – showing the extent of spread of the tumour.

p.TMM Post surgical histopathological classification.

P   An assessment of the P categories is based on evidence derived from surgical operation and histopathology, i.e. when a tissue other than biopsy is available for examination.

Pls   Pre-invasive carcinoma, carcinoma in situ.

Px   The extent of invasion cannot be assessed.

Po   No tumour found on examination of specimen.

Pl   Tumour not extending beyond the lamina propria.

P2   Tumour with infiltration of superficial muscle not more than half way through the muscle coat.

P3   Tumour with invasion of deep muscle more than half way through the muscle coat or infiltration of perivesical tissue.

P4   Tumour with infiltration of prostate or other extra vesical strictures.

G   Histopathological grading – which is a measure of the degree of differentiation of the tumour.

Gx   Grade cannot be assessed.

Go   No evidence of anaplasia, i.e. papilloma.

G1   Low grade malignancy.

G2   Medium grade malignancy. } see UICC definitions

G3   High grade malignancy.

765

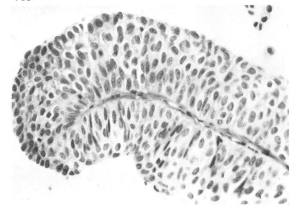

766

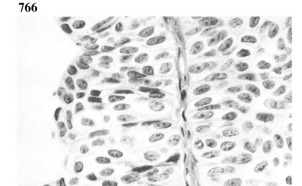

767

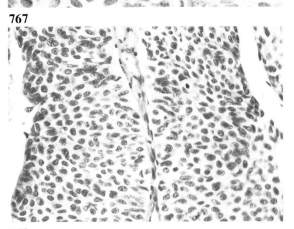

Histological examples of the various grades of tumours

Grade 1

765 **Papillary transitional-cell carcinoma.** This tumour has approximately seven layers of closely packed transitional cells covering a fibrovascular core. *(H&E × 160)*

766 **Papillary transitional-cell carcinoma.** Higher magnification of **765** showing the slight variation in size and shape of the transitional-cells. *(H&E × 256)*

Grade 2

767 **Papillary transitional-cell carcinoma.** This tumour has approximately 12 layers of closely packed transitional cells covering a fibrovascular core. *(H&E × 160)*

768 **Papillary transitional-cell carcinoma.** Higher magnification of another area of **767** showing the moderate pleomorphism of the transitional cells. *(H&E × 256)*

768

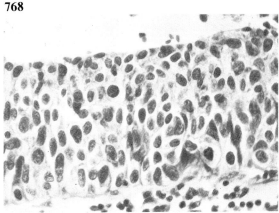

769

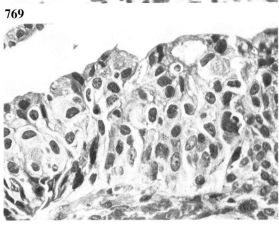

Grade 3

769 **Transitional-cell carcinoma.** These cells show considerable pleomorphism. It is difficult to tell that they are transitional cells. *(H&E × 256)*

Most papillary lesions in the bladder are papillary transitional-cell carcinoma. Lesions classified as papillomas show no histological evidence of malignancy.

Simple papilloma is only rarely seen. It is small with a thin stalk, usually single with very few fronds. Multiple bladder biopsies rarely reveal any additional tumours and the common presenting symptom is painless haematuria.

770

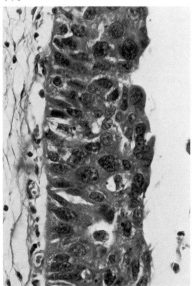

771

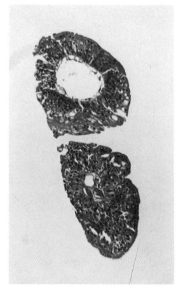

772

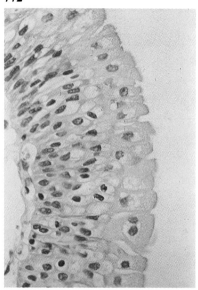

770 Carcinoma in situ. This is a section from a flat (i.e. non-papillary) lesion in the bladder wall. The thickening of the epithelium and the cellular atypia is such that it must be regarded as a carcinoma in situ. *(H&E × 160)*

771 Histological appearance. The simple papilloma is covered with normal transitional epithelium. It shows no atypia, thickening or mitotic figures. *(H&E × 26)*

772 Bladder. Section through a simple papilloma. Its structure is that of a simple finger-like outgrowth. This is a core of connective tissue covered with normal transitional epithelium. *(H&E original mag. × 256)*

773 Inverted papilloma. These uncommon lesions are usually recognised at endoscopy. Histology reveals their architecture which is that of a polyp with a smooth outer surface covering a mass of interconnecting trabeculae of transitional cells. *(H&E × 26)*

774 Inverted papilloma. Higher powered section showing the surface epithelium. These lesions appear to be benign but one has to be very sure one is not dealing with a transitional cell carcinoma. *(H&E × 64)*

775 Papillary transitional-cell carcinoma. Section through the fronds of a papillary transitional-cell carcinoma to show its architecture. *(H&E original mag. × 64)*

773

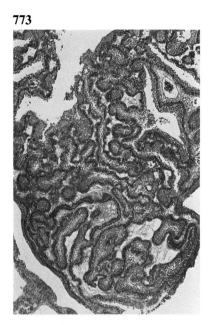

774

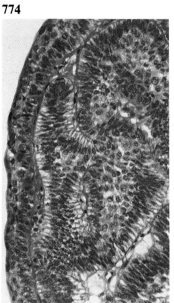

775

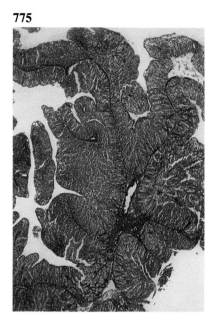

776 Urine cytology. Many a-typical transitional cells, some multinucleate, from the urine of a patient with a transitional-cell carcinoma of the bladder. *(H&E original mag. × 256)*

777 Urine cytology. Higher magnification showing the abnormal chromatin pattern in the nucleus of the transitional cells. *(H&E original mag. × 640)*

776

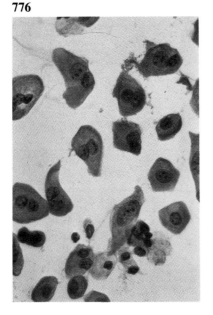

777

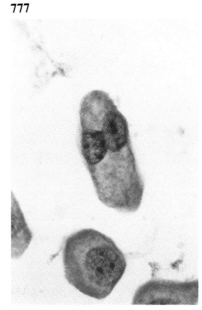

778a Discrete small-papillary T1 tumour with normal surrounding bladder mucosa. The fronded appearance can be seen.

778b A less well-confined low-papillary T1 tumour showing confluent appearance of this multifocal process.

778a

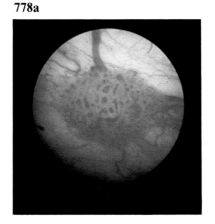

778b

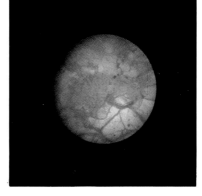

Haemorrhage close to a tumour is not infrequently seen and is due to trauma to a small vessel in one of the superficial fronds.

779a T1 tumour with a surrounding clot caused by haemorrhage.

779b A further example of a T1 tumour.

779a

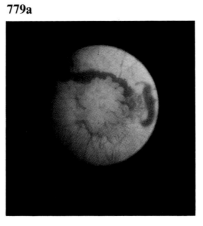

779b

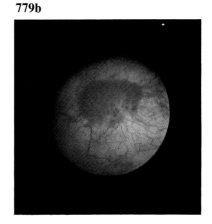

Histology of P1 tumour

780   P1 tumour showing invasion of lamina propria to be the deepest extent of the tumour. *(H&E × 256)*

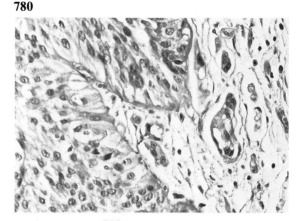
780

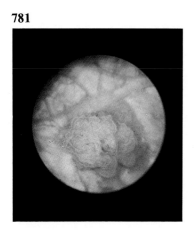
781

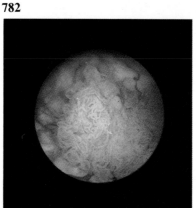
782

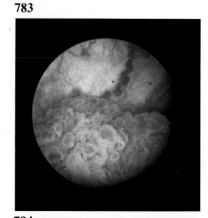
783

T2 tumours

These tumours may be small or large enough to fill the whole bladder. They may be round and tufted, showing short stunted fronds and have a broad base. Some have a wide pedicle which is difficult to see because of the exuberance of the tufts near the base of the tumour. Others have long delicate fimberial tissue up to an inch in length, which wave and swirl in the fluid medium like a bunch of seaweed. Sometimes the ends of the villae become avascular and their colour becomes either a pale yellow or glistening white.

781   A rounded tufted tumour.

782   Sessile tumour on the base of the bladder.

783   A similar tumour showing increased vascularity.

784   A typical long-fronded tumour. These tumours are large and it is always difficult to see the base, which may be very narrow.

785   Avascular tufts at the end of long fronds.

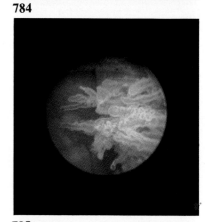
784

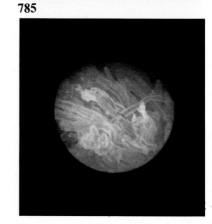
785

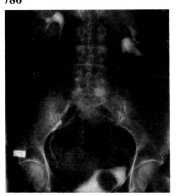

786

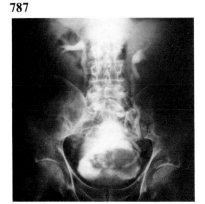

787

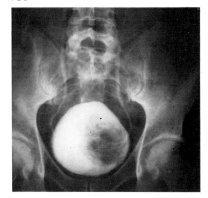

788

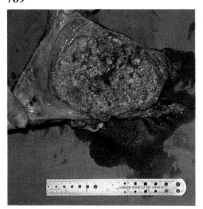

789

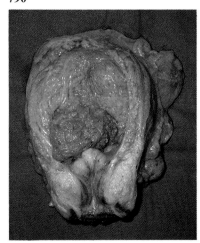

790

An IVU often gives valuable information.

786 IVU showing round filling defect in the bladder.

787 IVU of large superficial tumour anterior to the ureteric orifice, which is not involved, as the ureter is clearly shown behind the tumour causing the filling defect.

788 IVU of a large T2 tumour showing the villous structure and the absence of penetration as the bladder outline is smooth and regular.

789 Specimen of T2 tumour filling the bladder.

790 Large T2 tumour with a coincidental prostatic enlargement, especially the middle lobe. It has a wide base and when the bladder was intact filled a large area of the cavity.

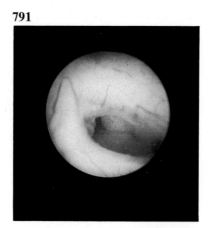

791

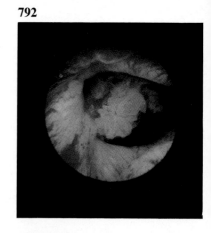

792

Bladder tumours may be one manifestation of numerous tumours involving any part of the urothelium. Multiple tumours of the renal tract occur in 10 per cent of all cases of bladder tumour. It is mandatory to undertake a careful examination of the ureter and renal pelvis in all cases of bladder tumour, and a bilateral ureterogram using a bulb catheter should be performed. On rare occasions bladder tumours may present at one of the ureteric orifices and have a thin pedicle.

791 Tumour appearing in a dilated ureteric orifice. Such tumours are small and move in and out with each jet of urine. Another rare presentation is at the bladder-neck.

792 Tumour involving the bladder-neck. Note the pedunculated base and the long fronds. Tumours which are seen in this area are usually one of many other tumours spread over the surface of the bladder.

Histology of P2 tumours

793 P2 tumour. Transitional-cell tumour invading the superficial muscle. *(H&E × 160)*

Endoscopic appearance of T3a tumour

These tumours are irregular, single and may have a surface slough. The presenting symptoms are haemorrhage, dysuria, frequency and occasional straining caused by superimposed secondary infection.

794 Infiltration papillary tumour with some superficial haemorrhage and necrosis.

795 Infiltration papillary tumour. A similar tumour with a larger area of surface slough.

793

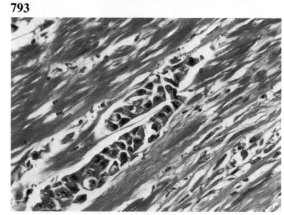

794

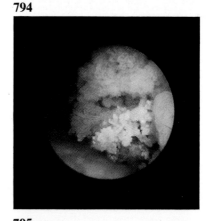

795

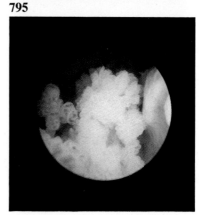

796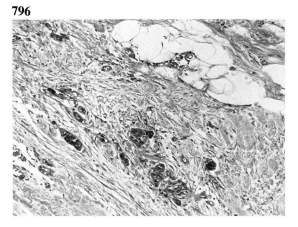

796a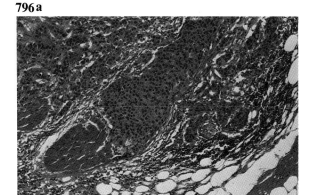

Histology of P3 tumours

796 P3 tumour invading deep muscle. *(H&E × 32)*

796a   P3b tumour showing invasion of perivesical fat. *(H&E × 64)*

Just as in T2 tumours an IVU is a great help.

797 IVU of T3a tumour invading muscle. The tumour involves the complete thickness of the muscle so that the outline is irregular.

797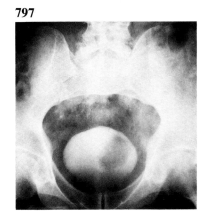

798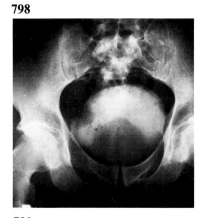

798 IVU of a small T3a tumour with total muscle invasion. This picture also shows a bladder filling defect caused by an enlarged prostate.

Endoscopic appearance of T3b tumour

It is impossible to differentiate between T3a and T3b on the endoscopic appearance.

799 Sessile nodular infiltrating tumour showing superficial necrosis, oedema and inflammation of the surrounding tissues.

799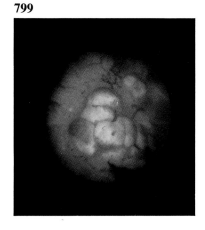

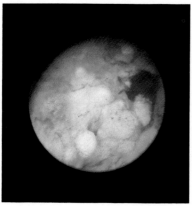 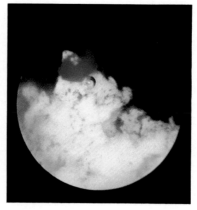 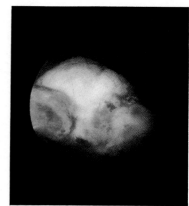

800   Extensive nodular infiltrating tumour with early ulceration.

801   Any T3b tumour can appear as a massive irregular growth with papilliferous formation. Here the villi are necrotic and ulcerated and appear as white almost transparent tissue.

802   A T3b tumour which is nodular, adenomatous and superficial slough. The brown areas are caused by submucosal blood pigment.

An IVU may give valuable information especially when there is involvement of one or other ureteric orifices.

803   804   805

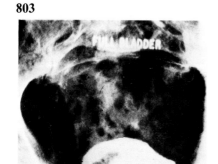 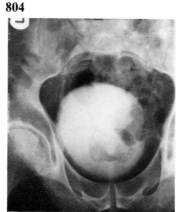 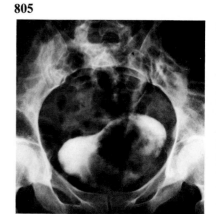

803   IVU of a small T3b tumour invading the bladder wall, where there is a complete gap in the bladder contour.

804   Further IVU of a larger T3b tumour invading the bladder wall.

805   IVU of a large T3b tumour. A large part of the bladder has been destroyed.

806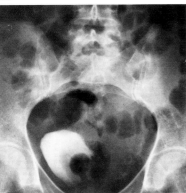

807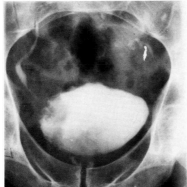

808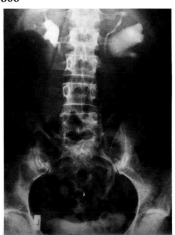

806   IVU of a large T3b tumour involving the left side of the bladder.

807   Multiple T3b tumours, one of which is involving the right ureter.

808   T3b tumour with early involvement of one ureter of a duplex system causing hydronephrosis. The upper ureter is involved causing dilatation of the lower renal moiety.

809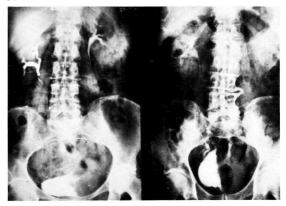

The intravenous urographic appearance may be a reliable method of assessing the invasive property of a bladder tumour.

809   A combination of two urograms, both showing extensive bladder involvement. One is a low-grade non-invasive tumour (T2), which has not affected the upper urinary tract, while the other is an aggressive invasive growth (T3a or T3b), which has caused a complete obstruction of the ureter.

810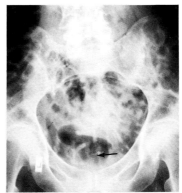

810   On rare occasions bladder tumours become calcified. An area of speckled calcification involves a tumour on the left side of the base of the bladder. This is usually a T3b or T4 tumour.

811

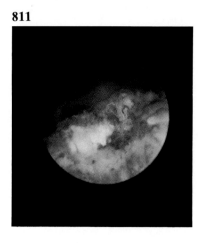

812

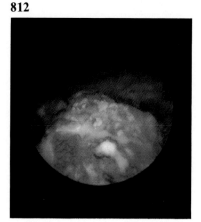

813

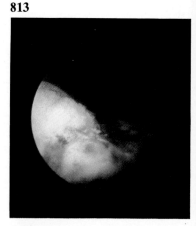

814

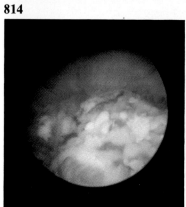

815

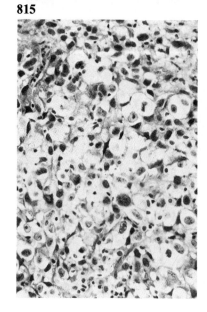

Endoscopic appearances of T4 tumours

The endoscopic appearances are indistinguishable from T3b tumours although the lesions tend to be more extensive and ulceration is more common. The following four pictures show all the characteristics, ulceration, infiltration, inflammation and oedema.

811   Irregular form, with an amorphous appearance on section. No normal mucus membrane is seen and on bimanual examination the bladder wall feels thickened and indurated with extension into the paravesical tissues.

812   Ulcerated tumour surface. There is superimposed inflammation, manifested by granulation tissue spreading on to the bladder.

813   Tumour haemorrhage. Some tumours have altered blood pigments on the surface, which implies haemorrhage into the tumour.

814   Tumour calcification. Another appearance is a white area caused by calcification which is well shown in this picture.

815   Undifferentiated carcinoma. This solid invasive tumour lacks differentiating features by which one can identify it as being of transitional-cell origin. *(H&E × 256)*

816

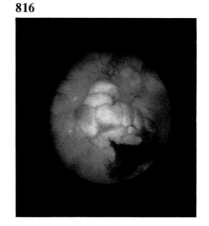

816 Undifferentiated carcinoma. The endoscopic appearances are indistinguishable from a T3a or T3b tumour, although the nodular appearance shown here is often seen.

817

818

819

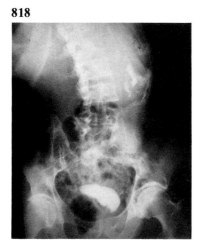

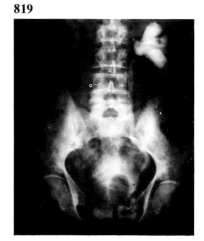

817 and 818 Undifferentiated carcinoma. An antero-posterior and lateral IVU of T4 tumour. The tumour was palpable and fixed to the pelvic wall. It may be difficult to differentiate between the T3b and T4 tumours by this investigation.

Advanced T4 tumours can invade surrounding bone

819 Undifferentiated carcinoma. IVU showing not only the left ureter involved but also there is destruction of part of the pubic and ischial bones.

820a

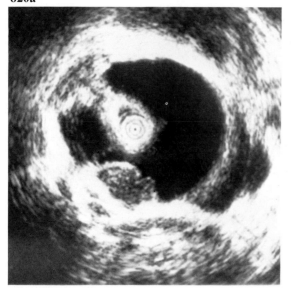

820b

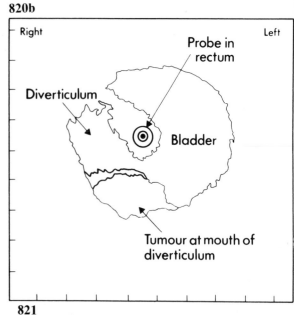

Right ⎯ Left

Probe in rectum

Diverticulum

Bladder

Tumour at mouth of diverticulum

820a and b   An ultrasound recording demonstrates an unsuspected tumour at the mouth of a diverticulum. With further experience staging of bladder tumours may be possible with ultrasound.

With diagnostic ultrasound, it has not been possible to achieve the complete diagnostic potential of ultrasound for bladder scanning. However, with recent developments it is now possible to introduce the transducer into the bladder through the cystoscope. The transducer head can be rotated through a 360° circle to perform a semi-real time scan. With this technique, an accurate diagnosis of different bladder tumours can be obtained.

821   Normal bladder outline.

821

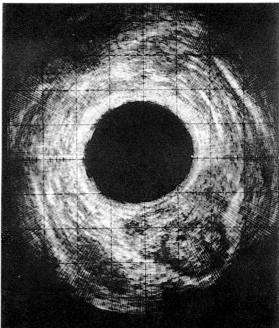

821a

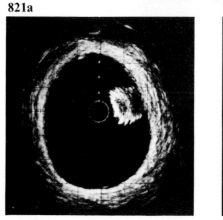

821b

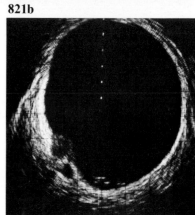

821a   T1 tumour.

821b   T3a or T3b tumour.

822a 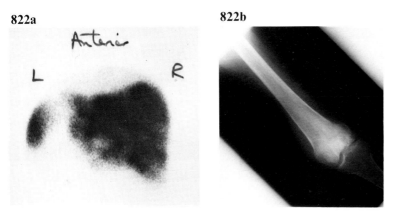 822b

823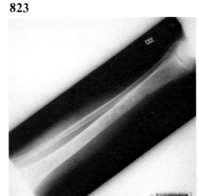

Metastases

As well as local spread the tumour can involve the liver.

822a **Scan of a liver** in which multiple metastases are present manifested by increased uptake of Tc99. Very occasionally bones are involved.

822b **Early metastases in femoral condyle.**

823 **Early involvement of the tibia in the same patient; lateral view.**

824 **Three months later, where there has been a rapid extension despite local radiotherapy to the area.**

825 **Histology of bone biopsy.** There are clumps of an undifferentiated malignant tumour scattered within the bone. The appearances are in accordance with a primary in the bladder. *(H&E)*

824 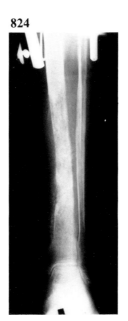 825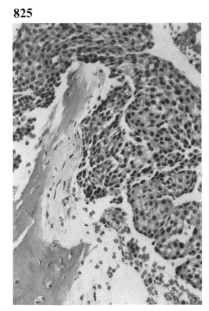

826

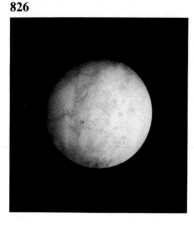

827

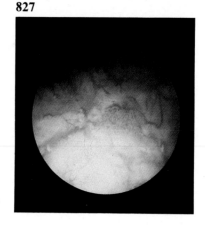

828

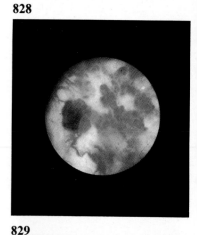

Local recurrence of tumours

Tumours can recur very rapidly and frequent cystoscopic examinations especially in the early stages and up to five years or longer are obligatory.

826   Early superficial recurrence T2.

827   Sessile almost confluent recurrent T2 tumour.

828   A more extensive recurrence with a superficial haemorrhage in one of the tumours, T2 or T3a.

829   A recurrence of a T2 tumour in the prostatic cavity, a TUR having been performed at the same time as the tumour resection.

829

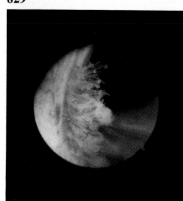

830

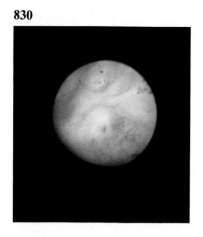

831

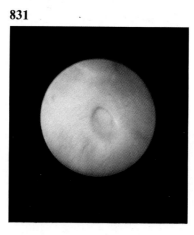

832

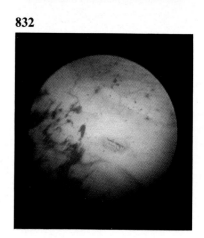

When the tumour involves an orifice, the orifice should be completely ignored at the time of the initial resection because not only is it often never seen, but it will invariably re-epithelialise. It is much more important to be certain that the tumour is completely resected.

830   Orifice in the middle of scar tissue.

831   A similar orifice flattened and rigid, but not obstructed.

832   Even when there is deep excavation of an orifice at the time of the tumour resection, regrowth of epithelium will recur although the orifice may be gaping and will probably reflux; a small price if the tumour is controlled.

Occasionally a tumour can start in a diverticulum.

833 A filling defect and an irregular external wall of a diverticulum caused by an extensive tumour. Often these tumours can be visualised through an endoscope introduced through the mouth of the diverticulum. Ultrasound may help to delineate the tumour (see **820**).

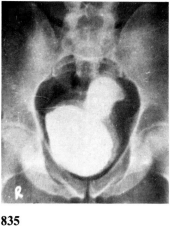

Adenocarcinoma of the bladder

Adenocarcinoma of the bladder is rare and usually arises from the dome of the bladder. Sometimes palpable as a suprapubic mass.

834a

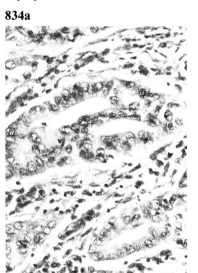

834b

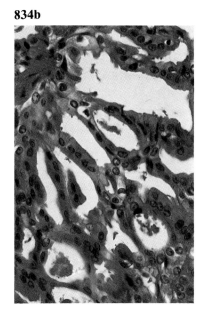

835

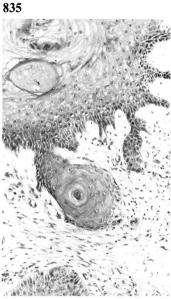

834a Histology of adenocarcinoma. This invasive tumour is composed of malignant cells making well-formed glandular structures. These are rare tumours and are particularly associated with urachal remnants and cystitis glandularis. *(H&E × 256)*

834b Glandular metaplasia may sometimes be seen in transitional-cell carcinoma. It must be distinguished from an adenocarcinoma. This section shows gland-like spaces in a tumour which is basically transitional cell in type. *(H&E × 256)*

Squamous carcinoma of the bladder

The transitional cell lining of the bladder easily undergoes squamous metaplasia, and many transitional-cell tumours show squamous metaplasia in some part of the tumour. However, the diagnosis of squamous carcinoma of the bladder should only be made when the whole of the tumour is composed of squamous cells. The endoscopic and IVU appearances are indistinguishable from the advanced T3a, T3b or T4 transitional-cell carcinoma; the diagnosis is made by the pathologist.

835 Histology of squamous-cell carcinoma. This invasive tumour is composed predominantly of cells resembling the prickle-cell layer of the skin. It is forming keratin and in the middle of the field a 'keratin pearl' is present. These tumours are particularly associated with stones, diverticula and bilharzia. *(H&E × 64)*

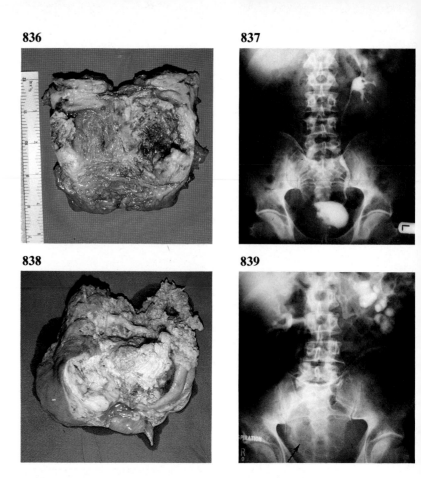

836 Cystectomy specimen of the bladder almost totally destroyed by a squamous-cell carcinoma, which has covered almost the whole of the mucus membrane. It is sessile, invasive and superficially ulcerated.

837 IVU of the same patient. The tumour fills the right side of the bladder and completely obstructs the right ureter.

838 Cystectomy specimen showing total destruction of the bladder.

839 IVU showing a thin rim of dye on the right side of the bladder. This was a huge tumour which not only involved the muscle layers, but almost completely filled the cavity of the bladder.

840 to 843 Industrial bladder cancer. Clinicians caring for patients with urothelial tumours must always be aware of the possible association with industrial chemicals, or even drugs.

Industrial diseases that have been accepted as a cause of bladder tumours are as follows:

People who work in a building in which any of the substances are produced, or used for commercial purposes.

1 Alpha-naphthylamine.
2 Beta-naphthylamine.
3 Diphenyl substituted by one nitro or primary amino group.
4 Any of the substances mentioned in paragraph 3 if further ring substituted by halogens, methyl or methoxy group.
5 The salts of any of the substances mentioned in paragraphs 1–4.
6 Auramine or magenta. This only applies to their manufacture, but not their use.

Chemical compounds have also been known to produce bladder cancer, and the two most important are:
Phenacetin.
Cyclophosphamide.

For practical purposes, the following occupations should be especially noted:

1 Factories manufacturing dyestuffs or pigments.
2 Factories engaged in textile printing.
3 Factories producing fine chemicals for laboratory use.
4 Rubber or electric cable factories.
5 Retort houses of gas works.
6 Rat catchers who use antu, which contains alpha-naphthylamine.
7 Laboratory technicians who use the chemicals for routine testing.

On a more individual patient approach, each patient should be asked if they have ever worked with chemicals in the rubber or cable industry, or in any gas works.

A tumour is initially suspected when abnormal cells are found in the urine, and these are diagnosed by means of microscopy. The carcinoma may spread to involve the uterus and vagina.

840

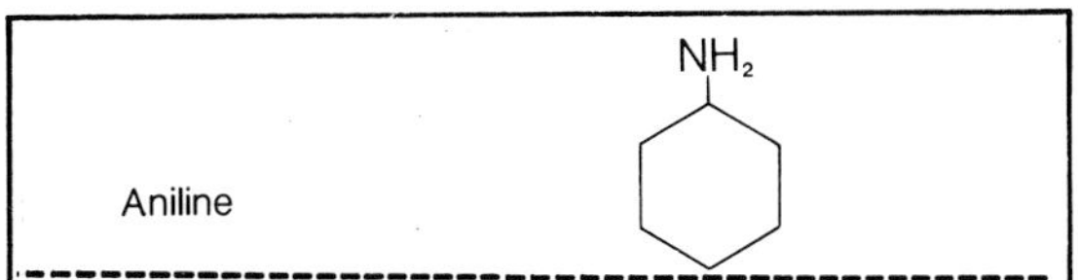

Aniline

841

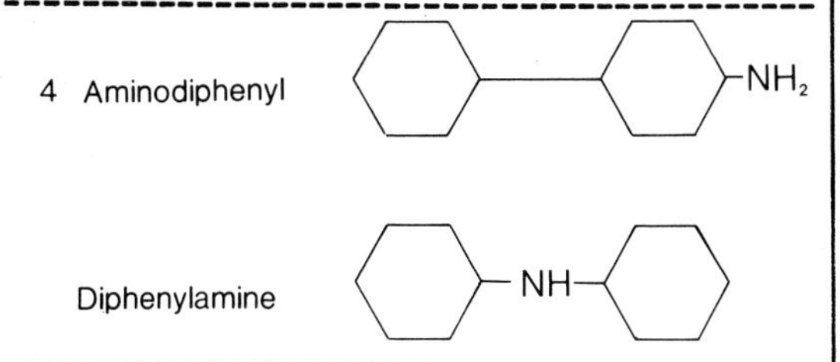

4 Aminodiphenyl

Diphenylamine

842

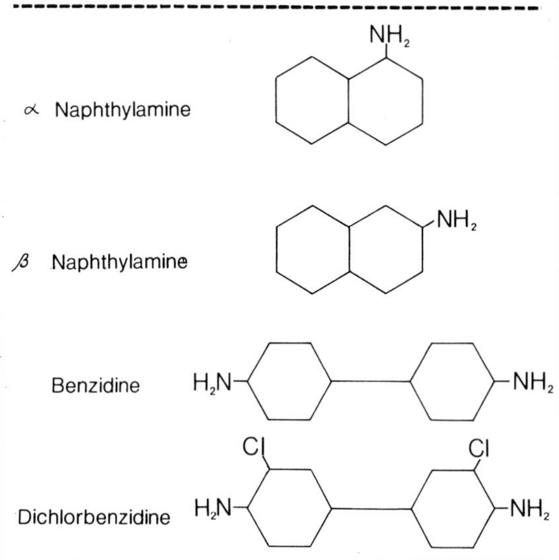

α Naphthylamine

β Naphthylamine

Benzidine

Dichlorbenzidine

843

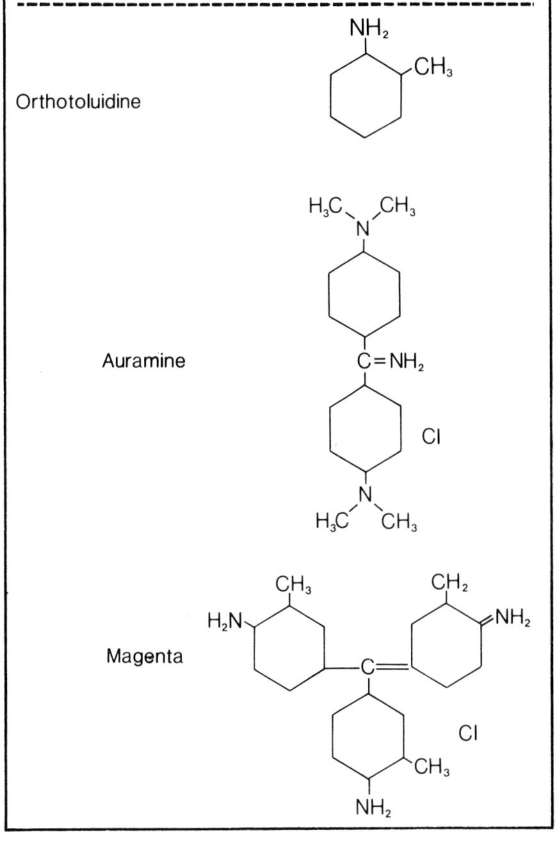

Orthotoluidine

Auramine

Magenta

844   Cystectomy specimen of carcinoma of the bladder which has involved the body of the uterus. It was a squamous carcinoma starting in the fundus which had invaded the uterus and the vagina.

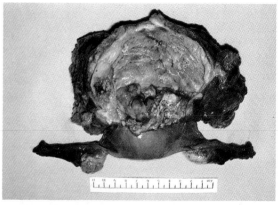

845   Cystectomy specimen of carcinoma invading urethra and vagina. Another squamous tumour which began at the base of the bladder and eventually ulcerated through the proximal urethra into the vagina.

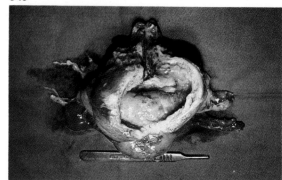

Unusual tumours

846   Phaeochromocytoma   (non-chromaffin   paraganglionoma of the bladder). The tumour is composed of nests of large cells with slightly granular cytoplasm. The nuclei are relatively small and usually centrally placed. Neurosecretory granules are present ultrastructurally. They are usually present beneath the epithelium in or near the trigone, probably arising from nests of persistent paraganglion tissue. Behaviour is usually that of a benign tumour but metastasis has been recorded. *(H&E × 256)*

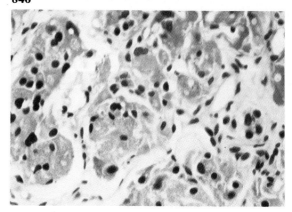

847   Rhabdomyosarcoma. This condition in the bladder occurs as embryonal or adult types. The type illustrated here occurs as a polypoid mass which is often oedematous and likened in appearance to a bunch of grapes (sarcoma botryoides). The polyps are covered with transitional epithelium, in the underlying tissue is an infiltrate of small cells which can be mistaken for inflammation but are malignant cells. *(H&E × 256)*

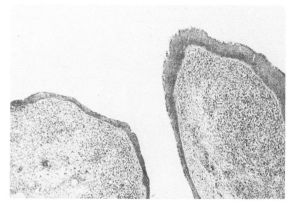

848

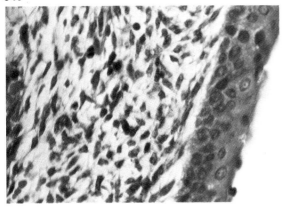

849

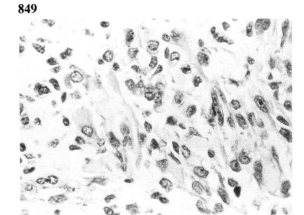

848 Rhabdomyosarcoma. Higher magnification of **847**, showing the oedematous stroma containing spindly cells. *(H&E × 256)*

849 Rhabdomyosarcoma. Higher magnification of **847**. Some strap-like cells. In the cytoplasm of some there are cross striations. *(H&E × 256)*

850 Carcinosarcoma. This is a biphasic tumour. On the lefthand side of the field is malignant epithelium (carcinoma), and on the righthand side of the field are malignant cells growing in a sarcomatous pattern. It is probable that the tumour is basically a transitional-cell carcinoma and that the 'sarcoma' is an unusual growth pattern of this tumour. *(H&E × 256)*

850

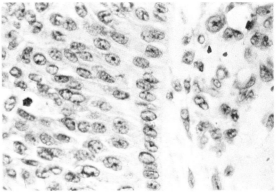

851

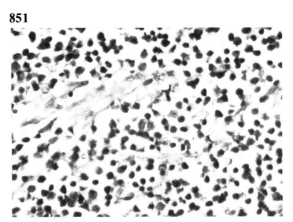

851 Malignant lymphoma. This may be primary or part of a systemic lymphoma. The tumour is composed of sheets of lymphoid cells. This lymphoma has the appearances of lymphosarcoma. It is important to distinguish it from reactive lymphoid tissue. *(H&E × 256)*

852

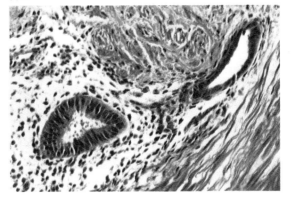

852 Endometriosis may form a tumour-like mass in the wall of the bladder. Histology shows two essential elements for diagnosis. First there are endometrium-type glands: second there are endometrial stromal cells around them. The bladder muscle is outside this. *(H&E × 64)*

853

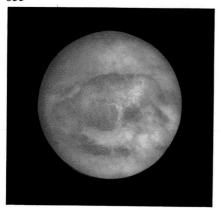

854

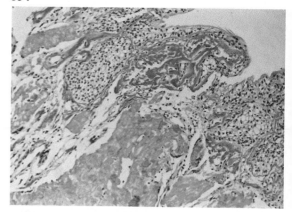

855

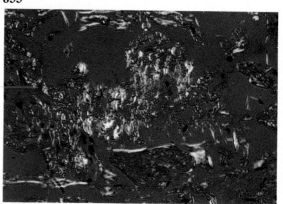

Amyloid.

853 Endoscopy reveals a solid vascular mass. Simulating a carcinoma and only distinguishable on histology from a neoplasm.

854 Section through a tumour-like mass of amyloid in the bladder. It shows a mass reddish material in the lamina propria, covered by transitional epithelium. *(Sirius red: × 64)*

855 Amyloid is a term applied to a number of abnormal fibrillary proteins. A characteristic which they have is that they stain with dyes like Sirius red (or Congo red) and subsequently, when viewed with crossed polaroids, are birefringent and dichroic. This section shows amyloid giving a green colour, while the collagen (which is also birefringent) is yellow. *(Sirius red: crossed polaroids × 160)*

856

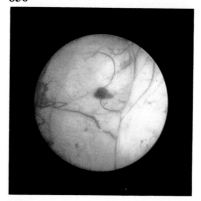

857

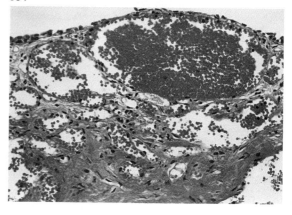

856 Bladder haemangioma. Small vascular malformations are occasionally seen in the bladder. The lesion shown here as a mucosal bluish mass, on histology proved entirely benign.

857 Bladder haemangioma. A haemangioma is a vascular malformation composed of thin-walled vascular channels lined with endothelium and filled with blood. In this section the attenuated epithelium (at the top) covers blood-filled channels of various sizes. *(H&E × 160)*

9 Diseases of the prostate

Diseases of the prostate and bladder-neck, together with urethral stricture (see Chapter 10) are responsible for the main causes of urinary outflow obstruction in the male.

Benign prostatic hypertrophy and bladder-neck obstruction

Benign enlargement of the prostate is a complex pathological process which tends to arise in relation to the central group of prostatic glands and may lead to urethral compression. However, the changes may be confined to the bladder-neck region, but either type of process may lead to outflow obstruction. The classic presentation of prostatism, hesitancy in initiation of micturition, a poor urinary stream, and post-micturition dribbling is often associated with nocturia. Occasionally haematuria and urgency may occur, and dysuria is found when urinary tract infection supervenes. The presence of residual urine encourages this complication.

858

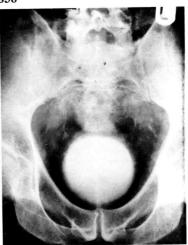

858 The post-micturition phase of the IVU shows residual urine and bladder-wall thickening.

859

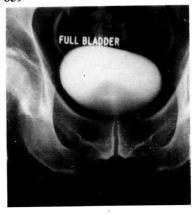

859 Prostatic hypertrophy may be observed by the presence of a prostatic impression in the bladder base, but this is an unreliable sign in assessing prostatic size.

860

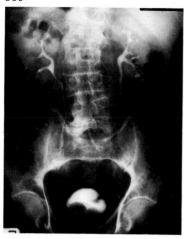

861

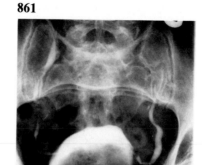

862

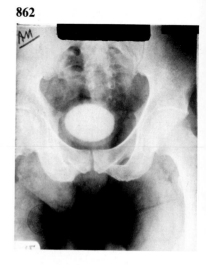

863

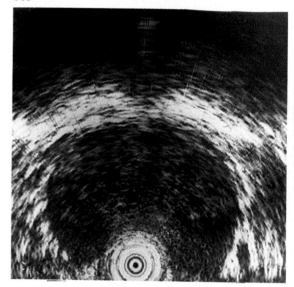

860 **When haematuria is a presenting symptom**, it must not be forgotten that bladder tumours do coexist; the filling defects of both a bladder tumour and benign prostatic hypertrophy are seen in this bladder film, underlying the need for cystoscopy in every case of prostatic pathology.

861 **A gross prostatic impression with ureteric hooking.**

862 **Bladder-neck obstruction.** In obstruction by the bladder-neck alone the bladder is thickened and spherical with no basal impression.

Ultrasound

863 and 864 **Typical scan of patient with benign prostatic hyperplasia** showing a rounded intact capsule and a homogenous parenchymal echo pattern.

864

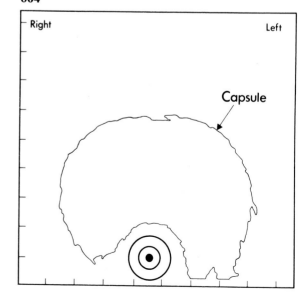

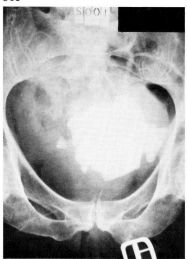
865

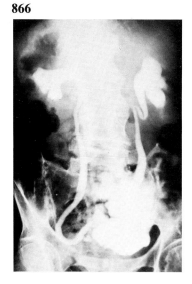
866

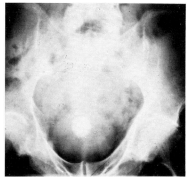
867

865 **Calculi may form as a result of incomplete bladder emptying.**

866 **The obstructed upper tracts with ureteric hooking,** particularly marked on the left side, are seen in this patient with the large, irregular bladder calculus.

867 **Phosphatic calculi** are frequently smooth and ovoid in shape.

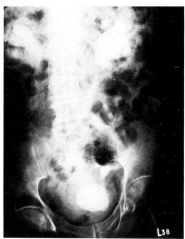
868

868 **Upper tract dilatation** is shown in this patient with a bladder calculus.

869 **Multiple bladder calculi** may occur.

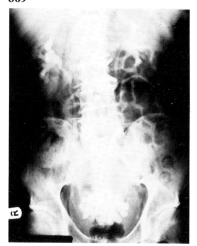
869

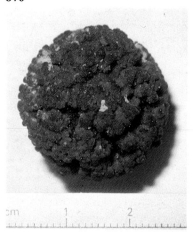

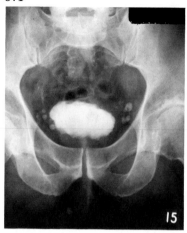

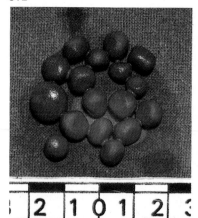

873

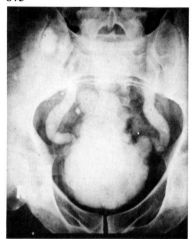

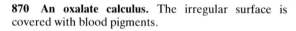

870 An oxalate calculus. The irregular surface is covered with blood pigments.

871 An irregular vesical base is seen in this patient with uric acid stones. The calculi are radiolucent.

872 Radiolucent uric acid stones after removal surrounded by blood pigment.

873 Classic bilateral ureteric hold-up with the 'fish-hook' deformity demonstrated.

874 Progression to bilateral hydronephrosis may occur with chronic retention and obstruction.

874

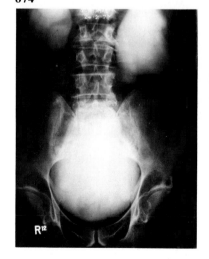

875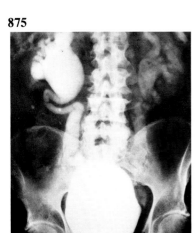

876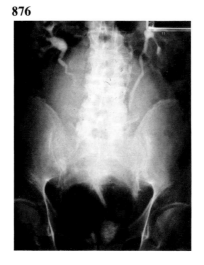

877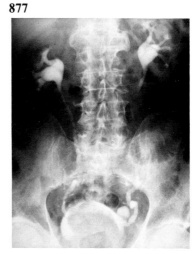

875 Reflux may also occur as seen here on the right side.

876 Chronic retention, here associated with gross prostatic calcification, may not affect the upper tracts which here are seen to be normal.

877 Enlargement of the middle lobe may be demonstrated as an intravesical filling defect. Note the normal upper tracts. It may be differentiated from clot by its smooth outline.

878 The vesical film of the IVU shows the middle lobe filling defect apparently unattached to the bladder base. A small left-sided diverticulum is also present.

879a and b Clot in the bladder shows two appearances of a patchy irregular filling defect not unlike a tumour.

878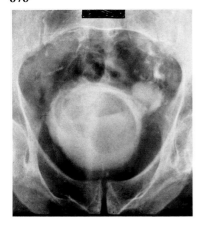

879a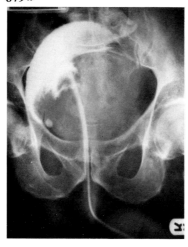

879b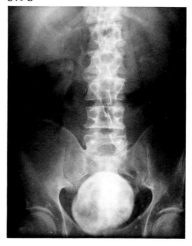

880

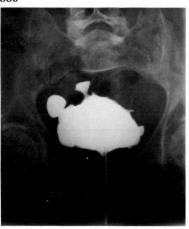

881

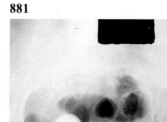
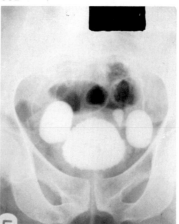

882

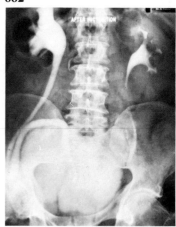

883

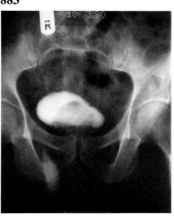

880 Multiple small diverticula may result from obstruction.

881 Two larger diverticula on either side of the bladder.

882 In this patient with a very large right-sided diverticulum the tortuous course of the right ureter is easily seen.

883 The bladder may also enter hernial sacs as a pseudodiverticulum.

884

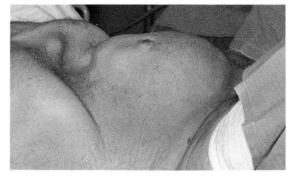

884 Retention of urine may be acute and painful or chronic and painless. The distended bladder is easily visible in the abdomen of this patient with chronic retention.

885

886

887

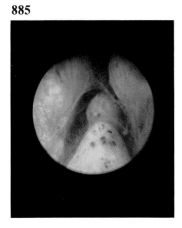

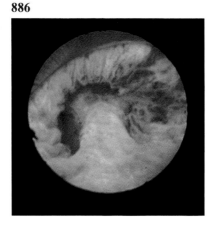

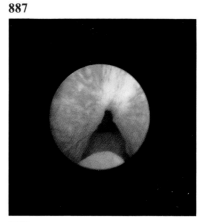

888

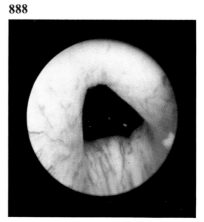

889

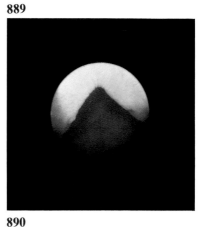

Endoscopy

885 Small pigmented lesions are frequently seen on the urethral crest.

886 Endoscopy is essential to assess prostatic obstruction and must always precede surgery. The veru montanum marking the prostatic apex is shown.

887 Moving through the prostatic urethra the lateral lobes are seen projecting inwards over the veru montanum.

888 At the internal meatus, a middle lobe is shown between the inverted V of the lateral lobes.

889 In the upper portion of the urethra at the bladder-neck, early lateral lobe enlargement is shown.

890

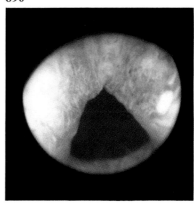

890 Increasing lateral lobe enlargement at the bladder-neck.

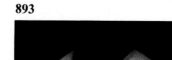

891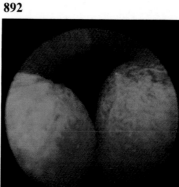

892

893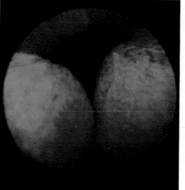

894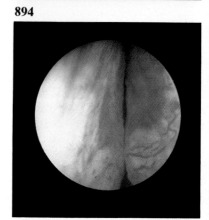

895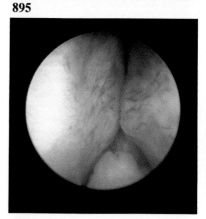

896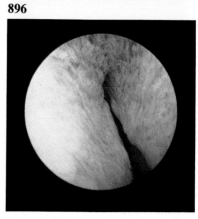

891 A narrow anterior angle with asymmetrical lateral lobe enlargement.

892 Bilateral symmetrical lateral lobe enlargement.

893 Unilateral enlargement of the left lobe.

894 The enlarged lobes meet in the mid-line.

895 **In the distal portion of the prostatic urethra** the veru montanum appears between the enlarged lateral lobes.

896 **Inflammatory changes** may be seen with injection of the vessels lying on the surface of the lateral lobes.

897

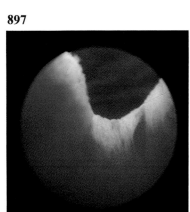

898

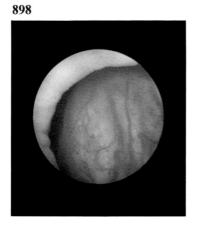

899

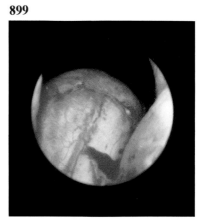

900

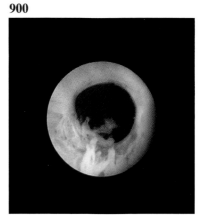

901

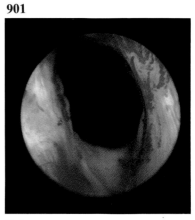

902

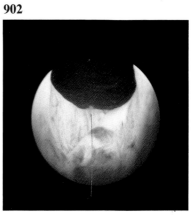

897 Inflammatory changes at the bladder-neck.

898 An enlarged and inflamed middle lobe.

899 A very large middle lobe.

900 **The obstruction may be caused by sclerosis** of the bladder-neck tissues.

901 Fibrosis may be marked in this process.

902 The crescentic appearance of the early obstructing bladder-neck.

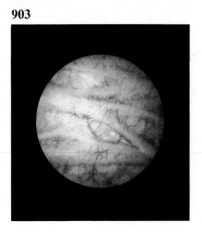

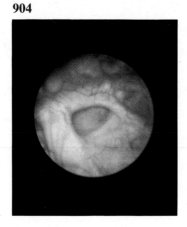

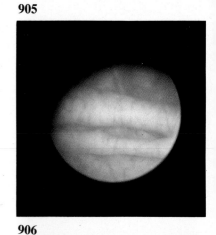

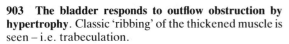

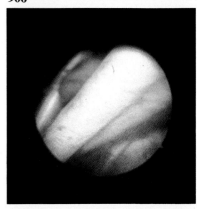

903 **The bladder responds to outflow obstruction by hypertrophy**. Classic 'ribbing' of the thickened muscle is seen – i.e. trabeculation.

904 **Increased trabeculation with early sacculation.** This may advance to diverticulum formation.

905 **Coarse trabeculation.**

906 **Very coarse trabeculation.** Note clot lying between the trabeculae.

907 **A shallow diverticulum.**

908 **The mouth of a large diverticulum.**

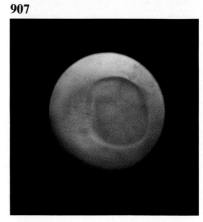

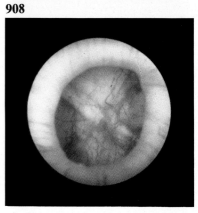

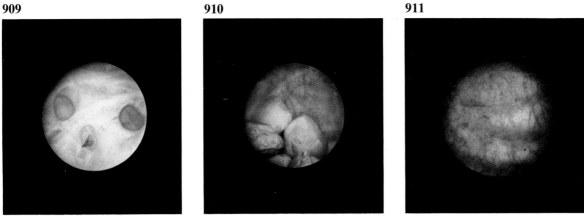

909 Multiple diverticula.

910 Calculi present in a trabeculated bladder.

911 **Urinary tract infection**, a consequence of residual urine and super-added infection produces cystitis and an infected trabeculated bladder results. Here the inflamed trabeculated bladder wall is seen.

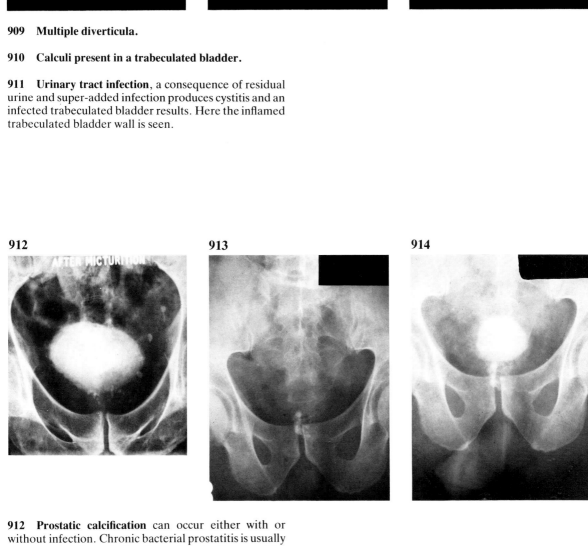

912 **Prostatic calcification** can occur either with or without infection. Chronic bacterial prostatitis is usually accompanied by calculus formation in the prostate. Here there is considerable residual urine with small prostatic calculi beneath the bladder base. Phleboliths (calcification in pelvic veins) are also present.

913 **A large prostatic calculus.**

914 **Post-micturition film showing residual urine** in this patient.

915

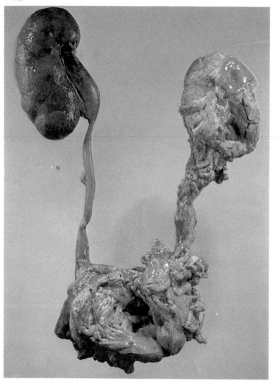

916

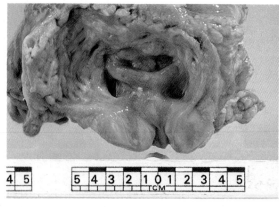

917

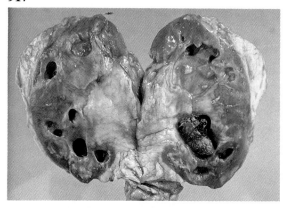

918

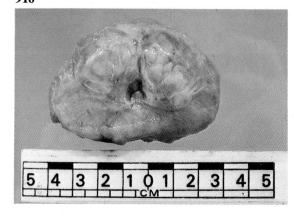

915 Effects of benign prostatic enlargement. A post-mortem specimen showing an enlarged prostate which has produced a trabecular bladder with multiple diverticula. There is bilateral hydroureter and hydronephrosis.

916 Effects of benign prostatic enlargement. A close-up of the bladder of the specimen seen in **915** showing the enlarged prostate with the thick-walled bladder distorted by muscle bands and diverticula.

917 Effects of benign prostatic enlargement. A close-up of the bisected left kidney seen in **915** showing the hydroureter, hydronephrosis and a stone in the pelvis at the lower pole.

918 Benign prostatic enlargement. A transverse section through the nodular enlarged prostate seen in **915**. In this condition the enlargement affects the periurethral portion of the prostate (median and lateral lobes).

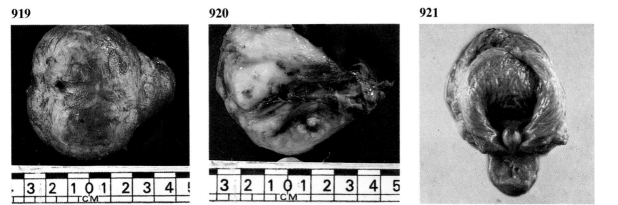

919 **Benign prostatic enlargement.** A surgical specimen of a nodular enlarged prostate.

920 **Benign prostatic enlargement.** Sagittal section through the specimen seen in **919**.

921 **Benign prostatic enlargement.** Post-mortem specimen of bladder and prostate illustrating median lobe enlargement and trabeculation of the bladder.

922 and 923 **Benign enlargement of the prostate** is caused by hyperplasia and/or hypertrophy of tissues normally found in the prostate. The major elements are glandular, muscular and fibrous tissue. Enlargement usually shows a mixture of these elements though one or other can predominate. Median lobe enlargement is often solid, with fibrous and muscular tissue predominating. Nodules in the lateral lobes usually have a large glandular component.

These two sections of a post-mortem specimen of prostate show the nodular enlargement affecting large areas of the gland. The trichrome picks up the fibrous tissue (stained green). *(Natural size: H&E and trichrome)*

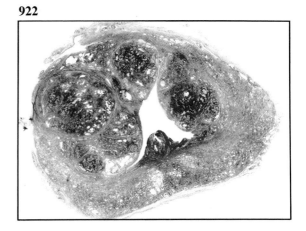

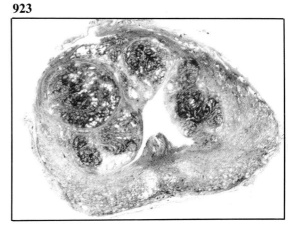

924

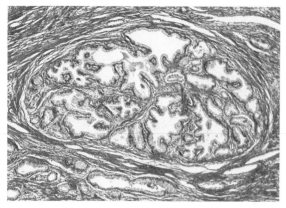

925

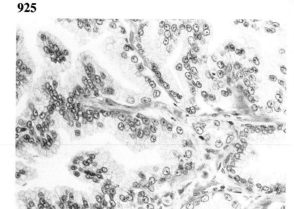

924 Adenomyomatous hyperplasia. A small nodule composed of glands, bands of fibrous tissue and muscle is arranged around it. *(H&E × 26)*

926

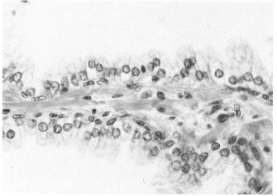

925 Adenomyomatous hyperplasia. Part of a nodule which is composed of hyperplastic glands showing papillary infolding of the tall columnar epithelium. There is little connective tissue between the glands. *(H&E × 160)*

926 Adenomyomatous hyperplasia. Higher magnification to show the epithelium of hyperplastic glands. There is a two-layered arrangement with tall columnar epithelium lining the lumen of the gland and a basal layer of cells lying beneath them. *(H&E × 256)*

927

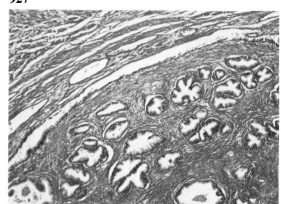

927 Fibroadenomatous hyperplasia. Part of the edge of a nodule which shows glandular hyperplasia but in which there is a much more prominent connective tissue component, which is predominantly fibrous. *(H&E × 26)*

928

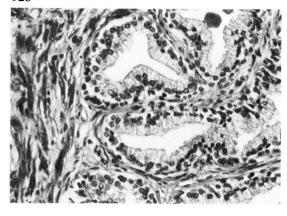

928 Fibroadenomatous hyperplasia. Higher magnification to show glands with smooth muscle fibres (red) and collagen (green). *(Trichrome × 160)*

929

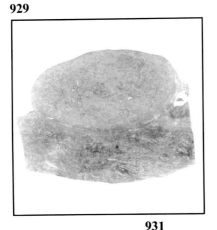

930

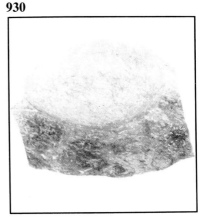

931

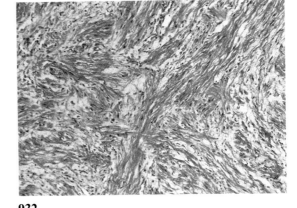

929 and 930 Fibromyomatous nodule. This solid type of nodule lacks a glandular element and is composed of varying proportions of muscle and fibrous tissue. Some small subepithelial nodules close to the urethra are composed of loose fibrovascular connective tissue with little muscle: such nodules are often called stromal nodules. *(Natural size: H&E and trichrome)*

931 Fibromyomatous nodule. A solid nodule composed of smooth muscle and fibrous tissue. *(H&E × 64)*

932

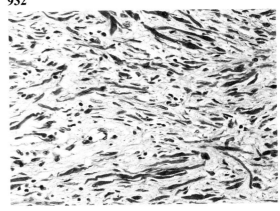

932 Fibromyomatous nodule. Similar area stained to show fibrous tissue green and smooth muscle cells red. *(Trichrome × 160)*

933

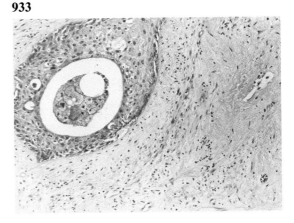

933 Prostate: infarct with squamous metaplasia. Occasionally prostatic nodules undergo infarction. Adjacent epithelium then often undergoes a change which makes it look like squamous epithelium. This section shows an area of infarction on the right side of the field. There is an inflammatory reaction at the junction of the dead and the viable tissue. The epithelium shows 'squamous metaplasia'. *(H&E × 64)*

Carcinoma of the prostate

In contrast to benign hypertrophy, this process usually arises in relation to the peripheral group of prostatic glands. Nevertheless, infiltration of the gland by the malignant process will produce outflow obstruction with all the radiological appearances shown in the benign disease.

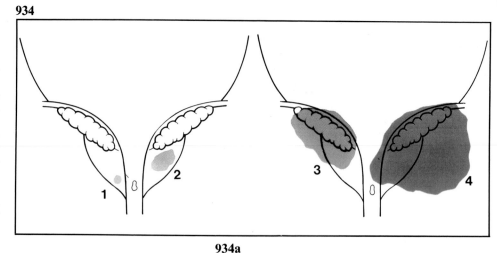

934

934 Diagram of the clinical stages of carcinoma of prostate. Clinically the gland may feel and look benign and the diagnosis is only made from the histology of the resected specimen. Because this process often arises in the periphery of the gland, biopsy by the perineal or transrectal route of palpable nodules may be required to prove the diagnosis.

934a Carcinoma of the prostate. Post-mortem specimen of a prostate showing a nodule extending posteriorly outside the capsule. The nodule and much of the prostate showed adenocarcinoma. The patient died with multiple metastases.

934a

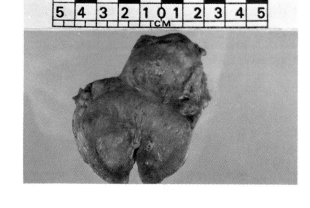

Ultrasound

935 and 936 Scan of a patient with a hard nodule palpable in the medial aspect of the left lobe of the prostate, but without any radiological evidence of prostatic calcification. Ultrasonically, an irregular echogenic area is seen in the parenchyma of the right lobe, typical of carcinoma or chronic inflammation. The capsule appears intact at all levels. Strong echoes situated in the medial aspect of the left lobe represent prostatic calculi. Histology confirmed a carcinoma of the right lobe.

935

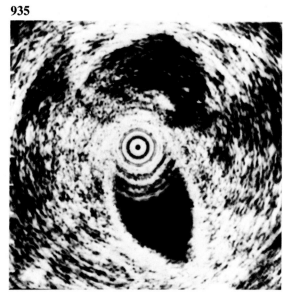

936

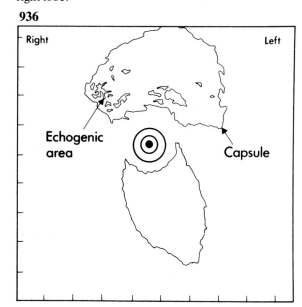

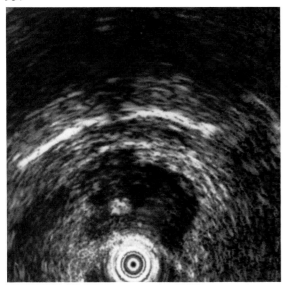

Right   Left

Capsular breach

937 and 938   Scan of a patient with digital findings suggestive of a confined (Stage T2) cancer of the right lobe of the prostate. Ultrasonically, there is a small irregular echogenic area in the right lobe with strong and middle range echoes. The right lobe of the capsule is distorted and anteriorly a breach is evident, suggesting extracapsular spread of the tumour.

939 and 940   Scan of a patient with a craggy hard mass in the left lobe of the prostate. Ultrasonically there were many echogenic areas in the left lobe where the capsule was indistinct but there was a clear breach anteriorly.

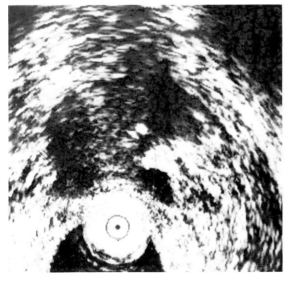

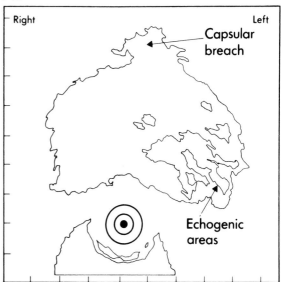

Right   Left

Capsular breach

Echogenic areas

941

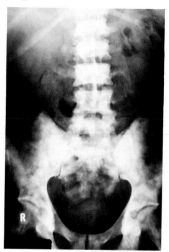

942

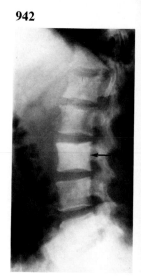

943

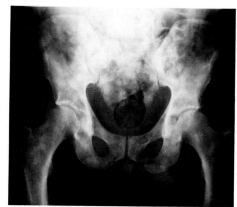

944

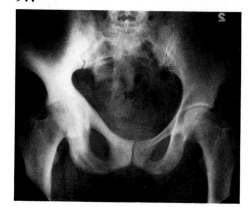

941 Carcinoma of the prostate spreads frequently to bone, particularly the lumbar spine via the valveless veins communicating between the peri-prostatic and peri-vertebral plexuses. Osteosclerotic metastases are usually diffuse and occur in 80 per cent of such patients.

942 A lateral view of the lumbar spine shows the body of the third lumbar vertebra to be sclerotic. A raised serum acid phosphatase (SAP) often, but not always, accompanies these bone changes, the formal stable 'prostatic' fraction usually being differentially raised to the tartrate labile fraction. Total SAP above 9.0KA units is strongly suggestive of bone involvement. Radio-immune assay techniques are now much more accurate in relating acid phosphatase levels to the stage of the disease process.

943 The pelvic bones are often involved in carcinoma of the prostate.

944 Paget's disease for comparison shows coarse bony trabeculae with expansion of the bone.

945

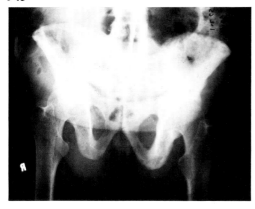

946

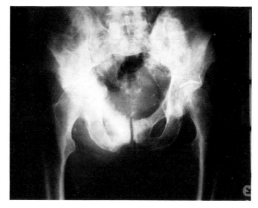

947

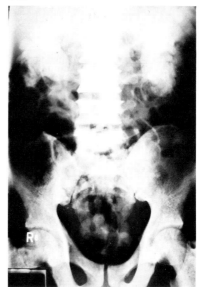

945 **Gross involvement of the left ischiopubic and iliopubic vami** are shown. Sclerosis but little enlargement occurs.

946 **The rare destructive form of bony metastases.**

947 **IVP showing gross bilateral hydronephrosis.** Marked density of the lumbar spine is seen.

948 **Widespread metastases in the ribs.**

948

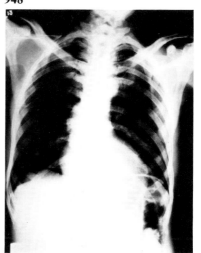

949

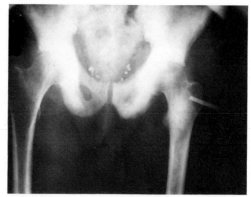

950   **951**

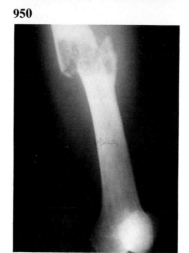 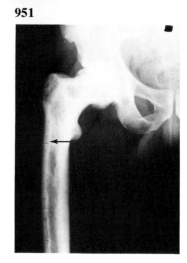

949   **Both the pelvis and left femur are involved with a pathological fracture** of the femoral neck.

950   **Pathological fracture of femoral shaft.**

951   **Paget's disease of the femur** showing bone expansion and bowing with a fracture of the lateral border.

Bone scanning by radioisotope techniques

Bone scintigraphy by Technetium 99 M (Tc 99 M) allows imaging of bony metastases shown by the increased uptake in the new bone provoked by the underlying metastases.

952   **Increased uptake in the ribs and dorsal spine.**

953   **Increased uptake in the dorsolumbar spine and pelvis.**

952   **953**

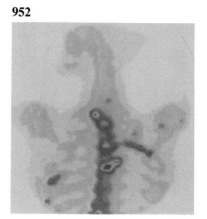 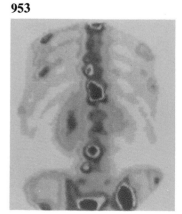

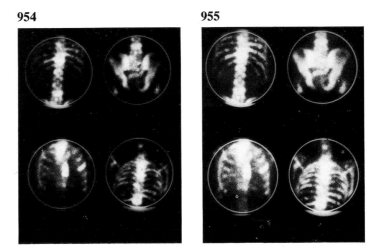

954 **Early metastases demonstrated by bone scan.** This may predate radiological change.

955 **Late generalised bony metastases.**

956a and b **Endoscopy shows the 'shaggy' irregular appearance of the malignant disease** process involving the lateral lobes and ulcerating the urethral surface.

957, 958 and 959 **The endoscopic appearance may resemble that of benign disease** in the early stages as the disease process begins peripherally and accompanying benign processes may have involved the peri-urethral tissues.

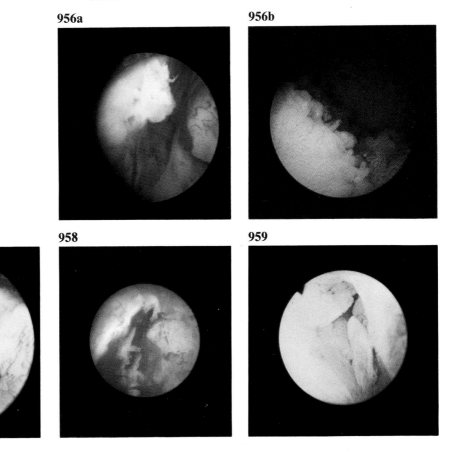

960

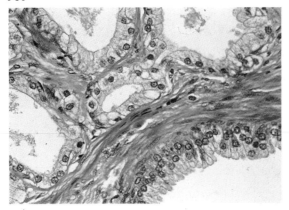

961

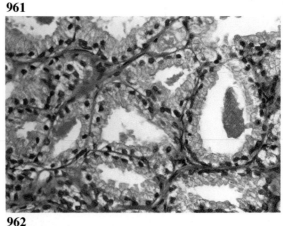

962

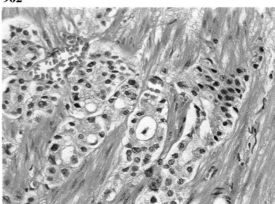

963

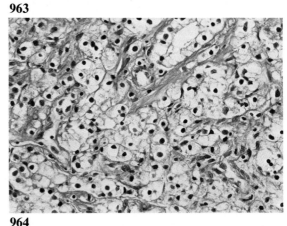

964

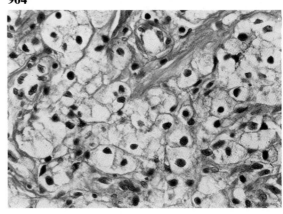

960 Prostate: atypical hyperplasia. Sometimes a glandular proliferation shows cellular atypicality without evidence of invasion. The glands in the upper part of the field show some abnormal features but carcinoma cannot be diagnosed. The term 'atypical hyperplasia' is widely used for such appearances; the significance of these appearances is unclear. The gland in the bottom righthand corner is simply hyperplastic. *(H&E × 160)*

961 Well differentiated adenocarcinoma of the prostate. Part of a prostate nodule in which the glands are small, rounded and lack myoepithelial cells. This is a well-differentiated adenocarcinoma. When such lesions are small, confined to the prostate and do not show un-differentiated cells, the outlook is good and treatment is not normally indicated. *(H&E × 256)*

962 Prostate: adenocarcinoma. A well differentiated carcinoma composed of well formed small glands which appear to be cutting across muscle. *(H&E × 256)*

963 Prostate: adenocarcinoma. Almost all carcinomas of the prostate are adenocarcinomas of varying degrees of differentiation. Other carcinomas (such as transitional cell and squamous cell) occur infrequently. Sarcomas are very rare. This section shows a moderately differentiated ådenocarcinoma composed of small acini crowded together. *(H&E × 160)*

964 Prostate adenocarcinoma. A higher magnification showing the nests of cells with clear cytoplasm and hyperchromatic, but not particularly large or pleo-morphic nuclei. *(H&E × 256)*

965

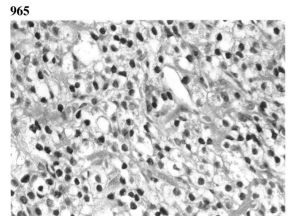

966

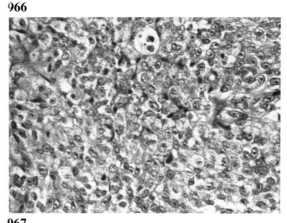

967

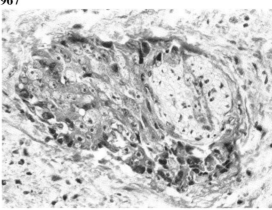

965 Prostate: poorly differentiated adenocarcinoma. In this tumour groups of tumour cells occupy most of the field but only occasional gland-like forms are seen. *(H&E × 256)*

966 Prostate: anaplastic carcinoma. This tumour shows no evidence of differentiation towards glandular or other epithelium. *(H&E × 256)*

967 Prostate: adenocarcinoma: perineural invasion. Adenocarcinoma may invade along tissue planes and is particularly likely to invade around nerves. The observation of perineural invasion may help in making the diagnosis of carcinoma in well-differentiated lesions. *(H&E × 160)*

968

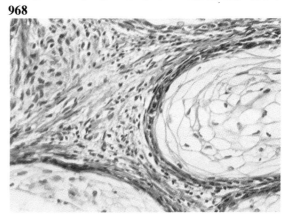

969

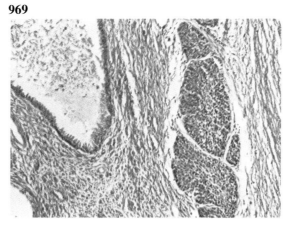

968 Prostate: adenocarcinoma: oestrogen treatment. Oestrogen therapy for carcinoma often results in the development in the epithelium of large pale cells with small pyknotic nuclei. This appearance resembles stratified squamous epithelium and is called squamous metaplasia. *(H&E × 160)*

969 Prostate: transitional-cell carcinoma. Transitional-cell carcinoma can arise in the prostatic ducts without tumour being present in the bladder of urethra. Such a tumour is seen here. There are normal prostatic glands on the left side of the picture while the solid clumps of epithelial cells have the appearances of a transitional-cell carcinoma. These tumours do not respond to oestrogens and behave in a similar fashion to transitional-cell carcinoma in the bladder. *(H&E × 64)*

10 Urethral inflammation, stricture, and tumours

Urethral disorders are principally inflammatory in origin. The male urethra is particularly prone to post-inflammatory stricture formation. Neoplastic lesions also occasionally arise in the urethra.

970 Urethral inflammatory disease may arise in the periurethral glands causing perineal abscess.

971 A paraurethral abscess secondary to gonorrhoea.

Urethritis caused by non-specific urethritis or gonorrhoea presents with urethral discharge and dysuria. It may be also associated with urinary tract infections.

972 Acute inflammation in the anterior urethra close to the glans.

973 Mild inflammatory changes in the penile urethra.

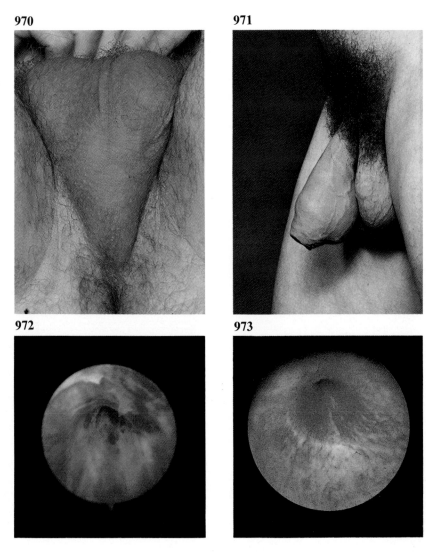

970

971

972

973

974

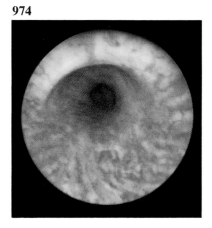

975

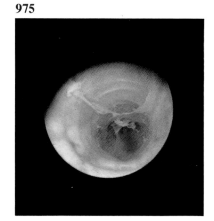

976

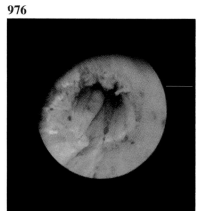

974 **Mild inflammation** in the membranous urethra.

975 **Inflammation superimposed** on a chronic stricture.

976 **Inflammatory changes** in the region of the external sphincter.

977 **Acute inflammatory changes** surrounding the verumontanum.

978 **Inflammation** involving the prostate and prostatic urethra.

977

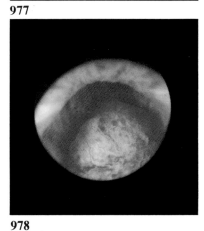

978

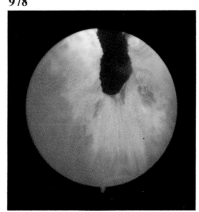

979 Congenital urethral diverticula may be found often presenting with urinary tract infection.

980 Large urethral diverticulum.

981 Ascending urethrography will demonstrate the diverticulum.

982 and 983 Urethral calculi may be formed in diverticula as shown here or may impact in the urethra having formed higher in the urinary tract. Occasionally a uretheral diverticulum forms after trauma.

979

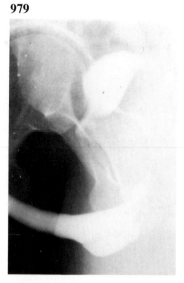

980

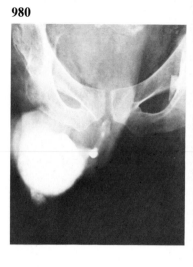

981

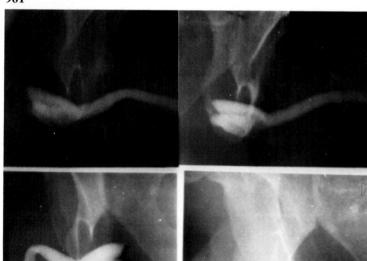

982

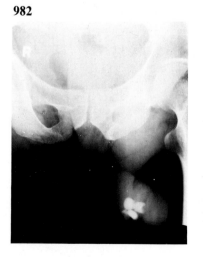

983

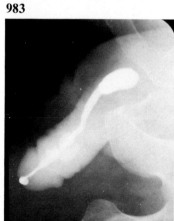

984

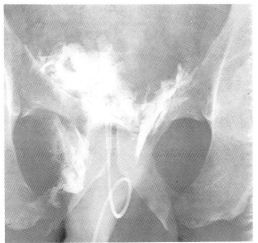

984a

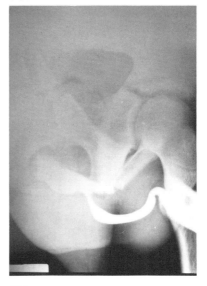

984 **Extravasation of contrast** in-dicates urethral and bladder damage. Note fractured pelvis.

984a **Trauma to the membranous urethra** frequently accompanies unstable pelvic fractures, when the perineal membrane becomes unstable and a shearing force is transmitted to the urethra. Bleeding per urethram strongly suggests this injury; ascending urethrography with water soluble contrast media provides the diagnosis.

985 **IVU showing elevation of bladder and medial deviation of lower ureter after urethral trauma.** Note fractured pelvis.

Fistula

986 **Endoscopy will locate the site of a fistula** in the rare situation when the urethra is involved in inflammatory or neoplastic disease. This followed a severe urethral injury.

987 **Fistulae may also result from long-term catheterisation.**

985

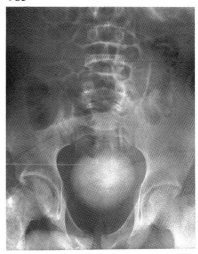

986

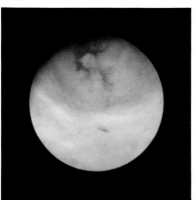

987

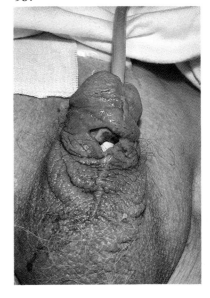

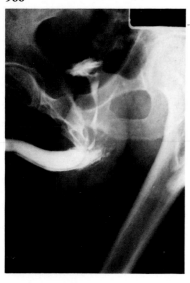 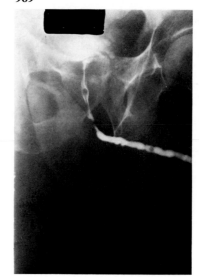 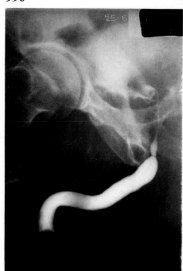

Urethral stricture

988 Urethral stricture caused by inflammatory disease or trauma leads to the symptoms of difficulty of micturition, straining to void, and a thin stream. Ascending urethrography will delineate the number, site and length of the strictures. When very tight strictures are present or there is associated inflammation, extravasation may occur.

989 Multiple anterior strictures.

990 Tight stricture at the urethral bulb.

991 Multiple strictures with associated diverticulum.

992 Stricture at the level of the veru montanum with false passage. These are usually iatrogenic after endoscopic manoeuvres.

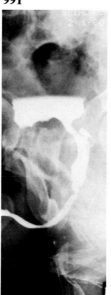 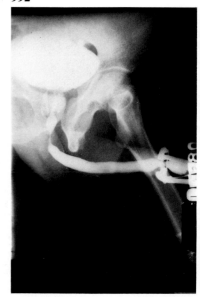

993

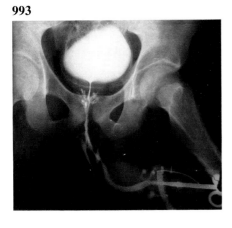

994

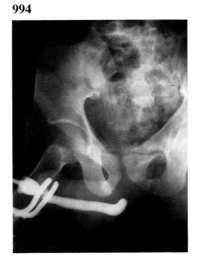

995

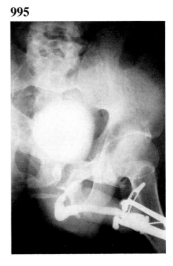

993 Double stricture in the region of the urethral bulb.
The prostatic ducts are filled here with contrast.

994 Complete obstruction at the urethral bulb. Note
the fractured pelvis.

**995 Complete dissociation of urethra and bladder after
extensive trauma.**

**996 Stricture with associated false passage after
bouginage.**

997 Stricture with a fistula distal to the stricture.

996

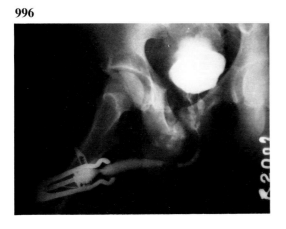

997

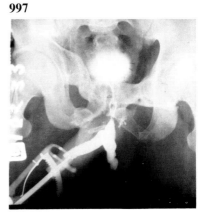

998
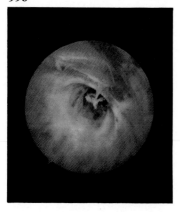

999
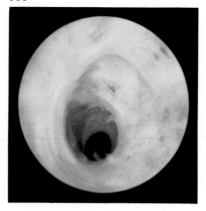

1000
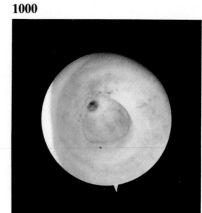

998   Endoscopy reveals the inflamed urethral mucosal appearance with the face of the stricture. The mucosa is seen to be inflamed.

999   The appearance of a scarred, fibrotic, longstanding stricture.

1000   A very tight stricture.

1001   A stricture with associated false passages.

1002   The healed chronic false passage in association with stricture.

1003   Operative appearance of the gross scarring in urethral stricture.

1001
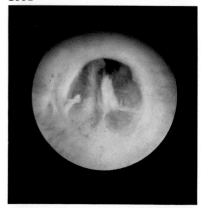

1002
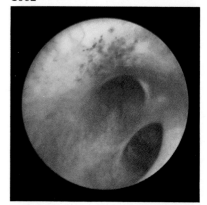

1003
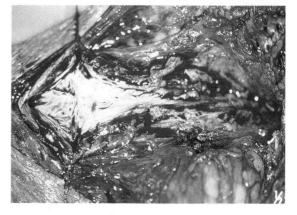

Urethral tumours

Urethral tumours are rare. Bleeding per urethram un-associated with micturition is the major presenting symptom. Viral lesions and occasionally papillary tumours are found in the anterior urethra and may protrude from within the external meatus.

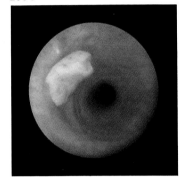

1004   Urethral tumour: benign endoscopy appearance.

Malignant urethral tumours tend to arise in the posterior urethra, and present with bleeding per urethram rather than haematuria and obstructive micturition symptoms.

1005, 1006 and 1007   Ascending urethrography will reveal an irregular ragged stricture in the deep urethra indicating a malignant tumour. These lesions are highly malignant locally, but rarely metastasise and so are amenable to radical surgery.

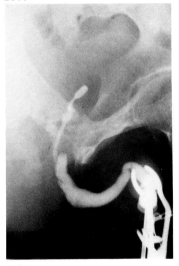

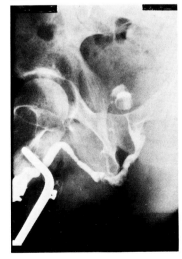

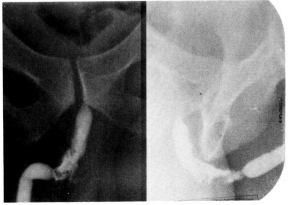

1008 Endoscopy reveals the irregular ragged appearance of a malignant tumour.

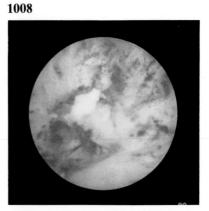

1009 The excised urethral tumour seen in 1008 is visible within the urethra.

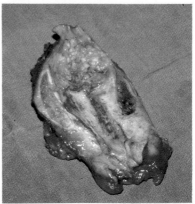

1010 **Transitional carcinoma of the urethra.** Tumour surrounds the bulbo-membranous urethra over a 6cm length. It is growing into the lumen of the urethra and is invading the root of the penis. Histology showed it to be a transitional carcinoma. There is also benign prostatic hypertrophy (median lobe) with evidence of bladder out-flow obstruction.

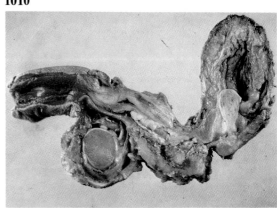

1011 **Carcinoma of the urethra** occurs extensively in local tissues without distant metastases. Here the lesion is ulcerating through perineal skin. This patient remains alive without recurrence three years after radical local surgery.

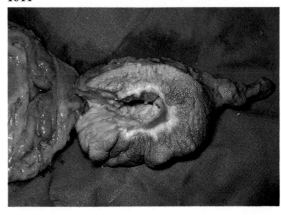

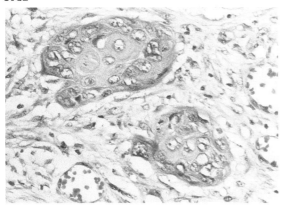

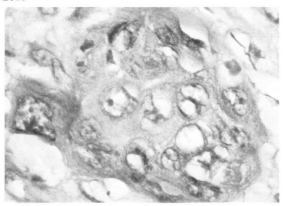

1014

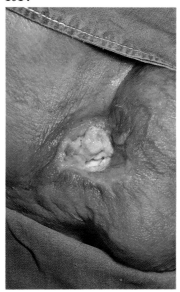

1012 Squamous-cell carcinoma of the urethra. The section shows islands of large cells, with eosinophilic cytoplasm and pleomorphic nuclei, infiltrating through connective tissue. Though it is not making keratin, the cells resemble those of the Malpighian layer (prickle-cell layer) of the skin. This is a poorly differentiated squamous-cell carcinoma. *(H&E × 160)*

1013 Squamous-cell carcinoma of urethra. Higher magnification of **1012** in which the desmosomes between some of the squamous cells are visible. *(H&E × 400)*

1014 The tumour grows extensively locally without metastasising distantly until very late in the disease process. However, fungation may occur through the perineal skin.

1015

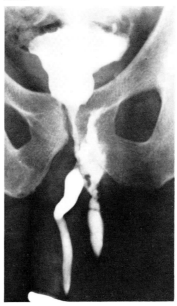

1015 Malignant fistula may occur in the urethra when malignant disease spreads locally from the rectum as shown in this ascending urethrogram.

1016 Female urethral carcinomata are also rare. This endoscopic view shows an early lesion at the bladder neck. There was no tumour lesion in the bladder.

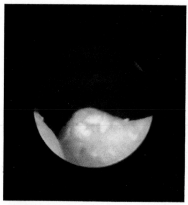

1016

1017 Transitional-cell carcinoma of the urethra exists in all the forms seen in the bladder. This tumour is part of a papillary transitional-cell carcinoma. *(H&E × 160)*

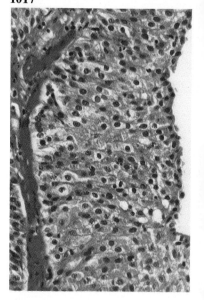

1017

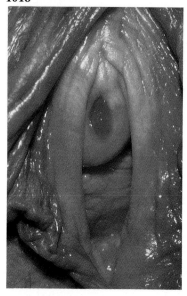

1018

1018 Caruncles are painful red swellings at the female external urethral meatus. They consist of inflamed, vascular connective tissue covered with epithelium. Often one or other element predominates, to give different histological pictures, but they are probably variants of the same process.

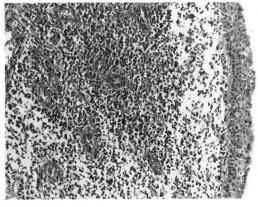

1019 A caruncle covered with transitional epithelium but composed mainly of loose chronic inflammatory tissue with blood vessels and a heavy infiltrate of inflammatory cells. *(H&E × 64)*

1020

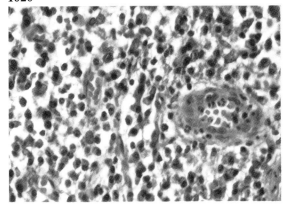

1020 Higher magnification of 1019 to show the cellular infiltrate, composed mainly of plasma cells, and one of the blood vessels with neutrophil polymorphonuclear leucocytes in its walls. *(H&E × 256)*

1021

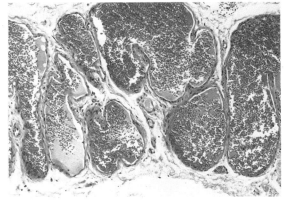

1021 Part of a caruncle composed largely of telangiectatic blood vessels and with little inflammatory cell reaction in the connective tissue. *(H&E × 64)*

1022

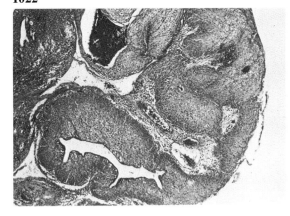

1022 Part of a caruncle showing marked epithelial proliferation dipping down into the connective tissue. *(H&E × 64)*

11 Penis and scrotum

Diseases of the penis may be classified as congenital, inflammatory, traumatic and neoplastic.

1023 The rare webbed penis.

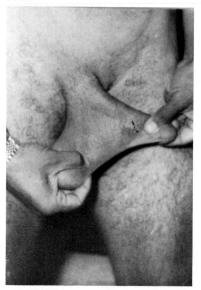

1024 and 1025 Balanitis. Inflammation of the glans penis usually occurs with an associated phimosis; the inflamed glans is viewed with the prepuce retracted. A more extensive lesion is shown in **1025**.

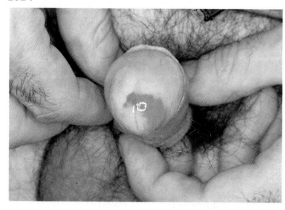

1026 The painless primary chancre of syphilis with its wash-leather base must be distinguished from a malignant ulcer.

1025

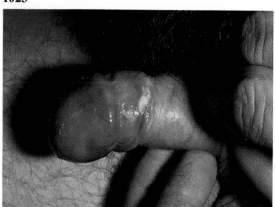

1026

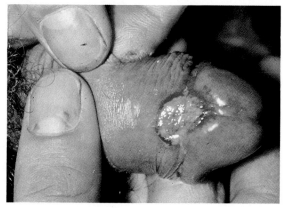

1027 Fungal infections may cause superficial penile lesions as in this patient with a monilial infection. The glans shows a mottled purple colour.

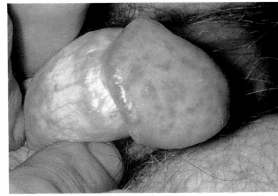

1028 Painful local ulcers with accompanying painful nodes occur in herpes.

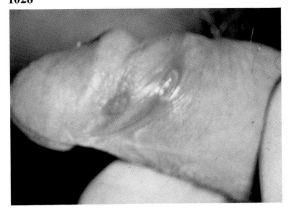

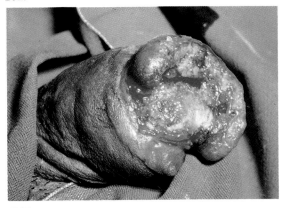

1029 Non-specific chronic inflammation may produce massive penile necrosis.

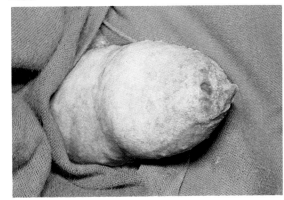

1030 Phimosis may be unaccompanied by infection but may cause mechanical pain with erection because of failure to retract the prepuce.

1031

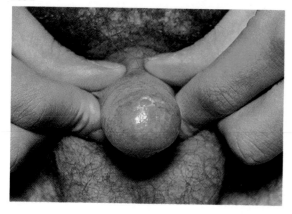

1032

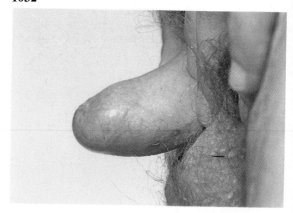

1031 and 1032   **A severe degree of phimosis** is shown in two views.

1033 and 1034   **Multiple papillary lesions** of viral penile warts.

1033

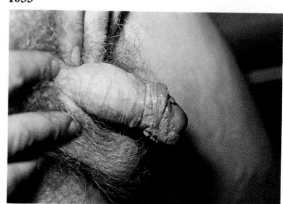

1034

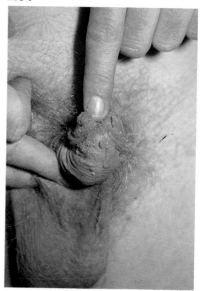

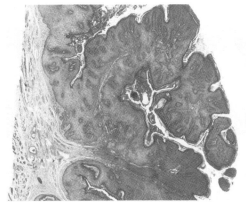

1035 Penile warts. Papillary outgrowths of hyperplastic stratified squamous epithelium. *(H&E × 64)*

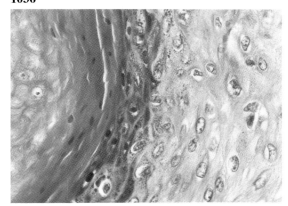

1036 Penile warts. A higher magnification of **1035** showing hyperkeratosis and parakeratosis (at the top of the field) overlying a prominent granular cell layer, with many cells containing keratohyaline granules and some cells being vacuolated. Beneath this zone is the acanthotic malpighian (prickle cell) layer. *(H&E × 256)*

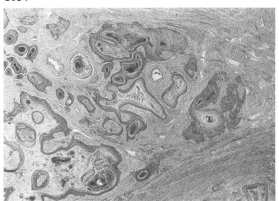

1037 Buschke-Löwenstein lesion. Occasionally large warty lesions are seen on the penis which grow into the underlying tissue and destroy it. The terms Buschke-Löwenstein lesions, giant condyloma accuminata, verrucous carcinoma and carcinoma cuniculatum are applied to such warty lesions which are well differentiated, which infiltrate but which metastasise late or not at all. Some authors claim that these lesions can be distinguished into separate entities, while others group them together as squamous-cell neoplasms of low-grade malignancy. This section shows islands of well-differentiated squamous epithelium which are keratinising and extending into the erectile tissue of the penis. *(H&E × 64)*

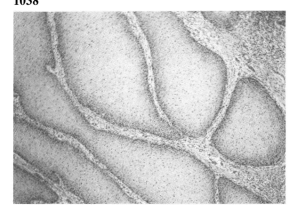

1038 Buschke-Löwenstein lesion. This section shows the pegs of well-differentiated squamous epithelium (this time non-keratinising) dipping down into the connective tissue. It can be very difficult to distinguish a benign lesion from a malignant lesion of this type. *(H&E × 256)*

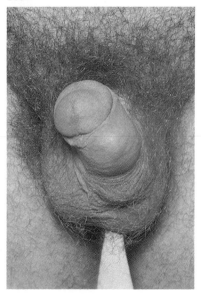

1039

1040

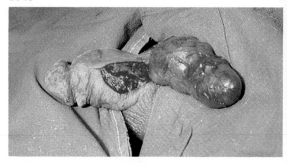

1041

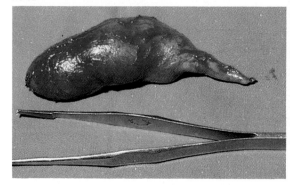

1039, 1040, 1041 and 1042   A dermoid cyst arising in the penile shaft.
Rarely do benign swellings develop in the penis.

1042

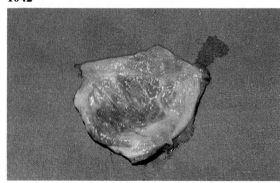

Ectopic testis

Occasionally the incompletely descended ectopic testis may lie beneath the skin of the penile shaft, producing the appearance of a tumour.

1043

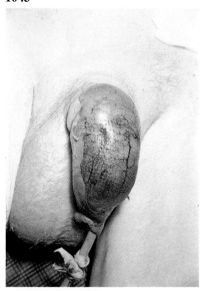

Gangrene of the penis

1043 Gangrene of the penis is very rare and almost always follows occlusive bands being placed around the penile shaft.

1044 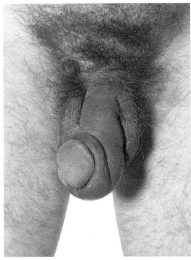 **1045** 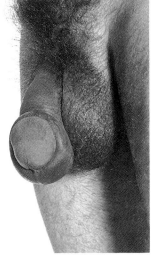 **1046**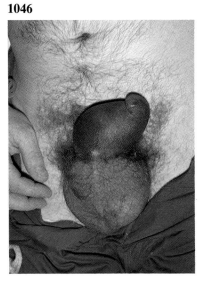

1047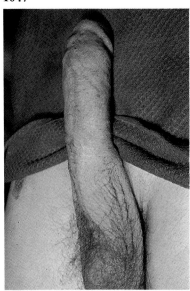

1044 Penile trauma, which is most frequently caused by coitus, will produce bruising and oedema with haematoma formation.

1045 If a corpus cavernosum is damaged, gross angulation may result.

1046   Intense penile bruising may occur.

1047 and 1048   Priapism, in which the penile corpora only remain persistently turgid, is usually idiopathic but may accompany haematological disease such as sickle-cell disease and leukaemia. The glans is not involved in the condition.

1049   Corpora cavernography shows failure of the dye to drain by the normal venous channels.

1048 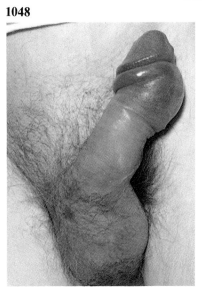 **1049**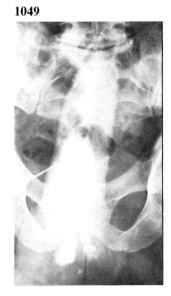

1050

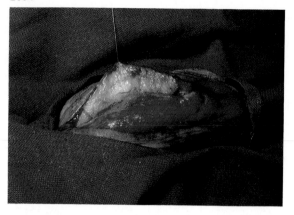

1051

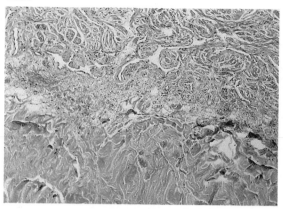

1052

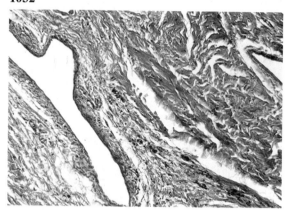

1050 Peyronie's disease is distinguished by the presence of painful, sometimes tender fibrous plaques arising in the walls of the corpora and leads to angulation of the penile shafts on erection. A plaque is demonstrated at surgery.

1051 Peyronie's disease. In this form of fibromatosis, proliferation of fibrous tissue (in the bottom area of the field) leads to obliteration of vessels and the development of a fibrous plaque in the corpora cavernosa. *(H&E × 26)*

1052 Peyronie's disease. The section shows the vascular channels of the corpora cavernosa being surrounded by dense fibrous tissue (stained green) and being obliterated. *(Masson's trichrome original mag. × 64)*

1053 Paraphimosis usually presents acutely when the retracted foreskin is not replaced and oedema is caused by the tight pre-coronal band.

1054 Paraphimosis. The condition is best seen in the lateral view. The tight band is clearly visible.

1053

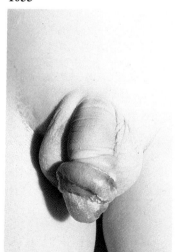

1054

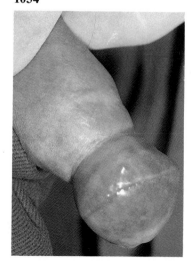

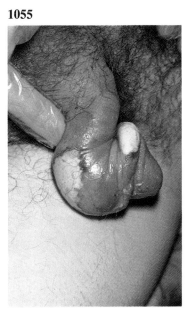 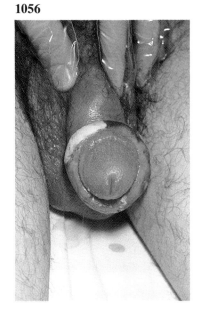 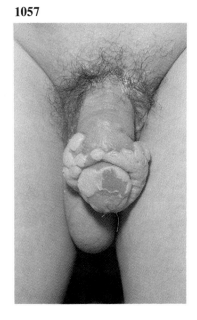

1055 and **1056** **Paraphimosis.** The condition may become chronic, causing severe local inflammation.

1057 **Warty-like inflammatory changes occur** when unsatisfactory long term penile appliances are worn.

Balanitis xerotica obliterans is a dyskeratosis of the penis, which is manifested by inflammatory changes, which in the very long term may become fibrotic and atrophic, leading to stenotic lesions of the distal urethra and occasionally progress to carcinoma.

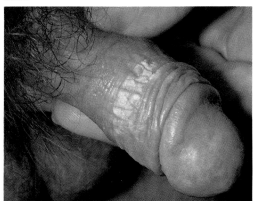

1058 **The rugose, whitish appearance of the retracted prepuce.**

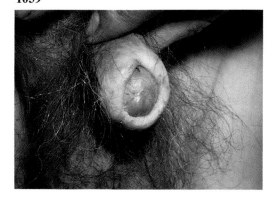

1059 **The stenosing band at the edge of the foreskin.**

1060

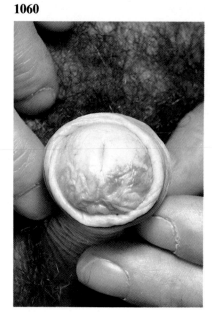

1061

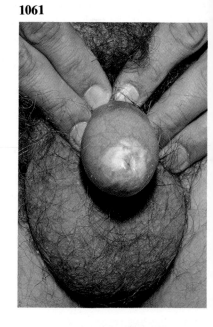

1060 Early telangectasia of the glans with the rugose glandular appearance.

1061 Atrophic changes around the external meatus lead to stenosis.

1062

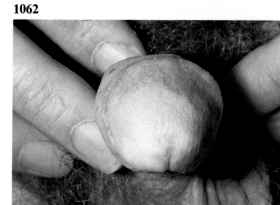

1062 Late atrophic changes in the glans.

1063

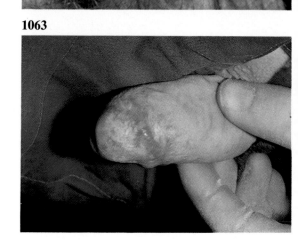

1063 Very late changes of gross telangectasia and coronal obliteration.

1064

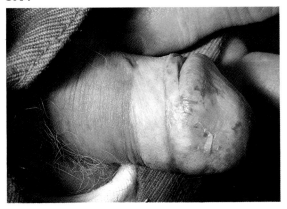

1065

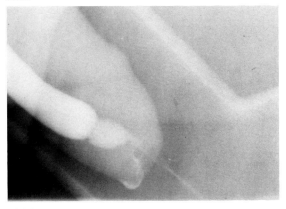

1064   Similar changes with a white preputial band.

1065   Urethrogram showing distal urethral and meatal stenosis.

1066

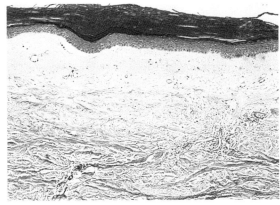

1066   **Balanitis xerotica obliterans.** Histologically this condition is the same as lichen sclerosus et atrophicus. There is hyperkeratosis, atrophy of the malpighian (prickle cell) layer of the epithelium, loss of the rete ridges and presence of a hyalinised band of collagen beneath the epithelium. *(H&E × 64)*

1067

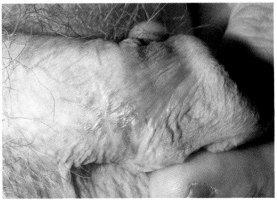

1067   **Carcinoma in situ lesions** include Paget's disease of the penis and the erythroplasia of Queyrat. The indolent slightly raised erythematous patches of Paget's disease can be seen.

1068

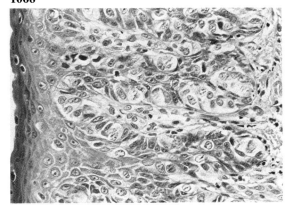

1068   **Paget's disease** occurs rarely on the penis giving a histological appearance similar to that in the nipple. In the epithelium there is widespread infiltration of the basal layer and adjacent layers of the epithelium with large cells with pale cytoplasm – Paget's cells. *(H&E × 160)*

1069

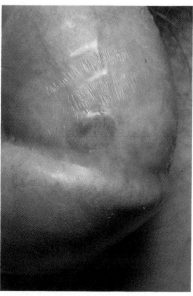

1070

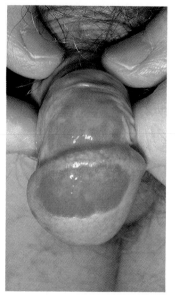

1071

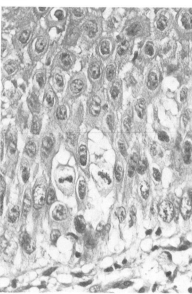

1072

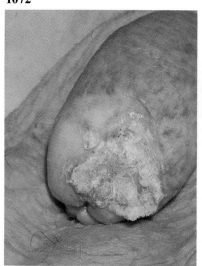

1073

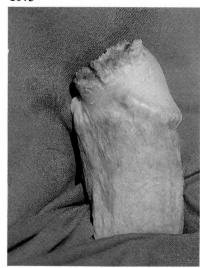

1069 Queyrat's erythroplasia. Persistent areas of reddened skin which are resistant to local treatment raise the possibility of such diagnoses, which can only be proved by biopsy. *(H&E original mag. × 80)*

1070 Very extensive Queyrat's erythroplasia.

1071 Queyrat's erythroplasia. The histological appearance of Queyrat's erythroplasia is that of a thickened dysplastic epithelium with cellular atypia and prominent mitoses. Infiltrating squamous-cell carcinoma develops in about 10 per cent of cases. The appearances are similar to Bowen's disease. Histologically it may not be possible to distinguish them with certainty. Bowen's disease is associated with other malignancies, whereas Queyrat's is not. Bowen's disease may occur on the shaft whereas Queyrat's is usually on the glans and prepuce. *(H&E × 256)*

1072 Horns of keratin may arise on the glans penis. This condition of hyperkeratosis is premalignant.

1073 The glans may sometimes produce bizarre forms of tissue.

1074 and 1075 Examples of penile horn.

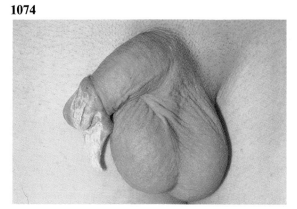

1074

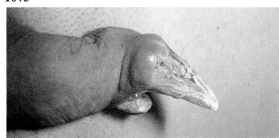

1075

1076 Penile horn. The section shows hyperkeratosis, parakeratosis and acanthosis. There is little atypicality of the epithelial cells. *(H&E × 64)*

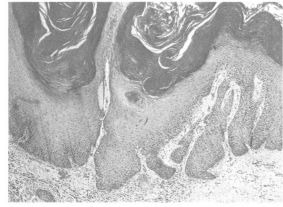

1076

1077 and 1078 Penile horn going on to a frank carcinoma in the same patient of a two-year period.

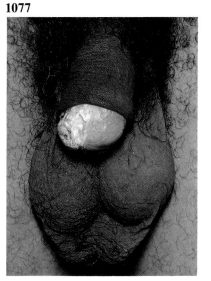

1077

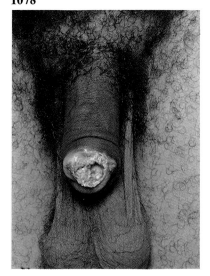

1078

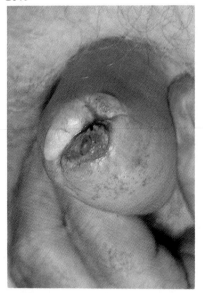
1079

Tumours of the penis and prepuce

1079 Carcinomata may arise from the undersurface of the prepuce and present growing from beneath it.

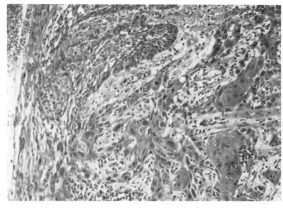
1080

1080 Prepuce: squamous carcinoma. The irregular squamous epithelium of the surface is on the left. Disordered strands of epithelium are invading down into the connective tissue. *(H&E × 64)*

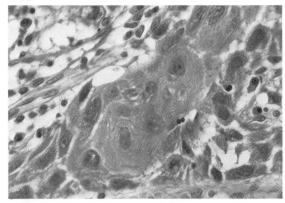
1081

1081 Prepuce: squamous carcinoma. A higher magnification of part of **1080** showing an irregular island of squamous epithelium in connective tissue, with a few associated chronic inflammatory cells. *(H&E × 256)*

1082 Penile carcinoma. When a purulent or sanguino-purulent discharge occurs from beneath the phimosed prepuce of the adult, then circumcision may be necessary to reveal the underlying penile carcinoma.

Stages of penile carcinomata

1083 An early lesion.

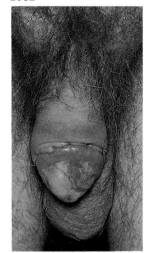
1082

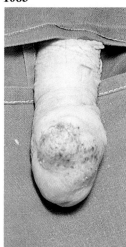
1083

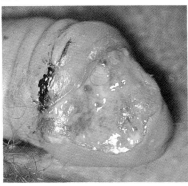

1084

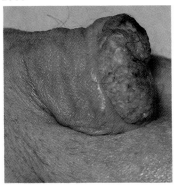

1085

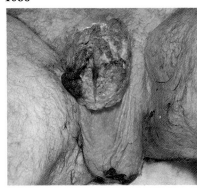

1086

1084 Local·destruction of glans.

1085 Bulky lesion involving the shaft.

1086 Erosion of the corpora may lead to torrential hae-morrhage as in this patient.

1087 Gross destruction of the whole penile shaft and involving the scrotum.

1087

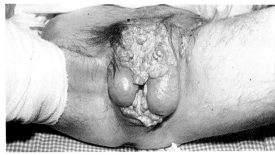

1088

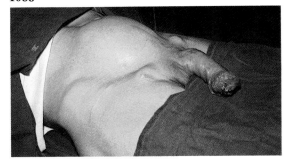

1088 Penile carcinoma. In the elderly, slow progression, fear and neglect, may lead to patients failing to present with penile carcinomas until they go into acute urinary retention as can be seen here. Groin gland metastases are well shown here.

1088a Scrotal wart.

1088b Histology of a wart. Papillary out-growths of acanthotic stratified squamous epithelium showing no evidence of malignancy.

1088a

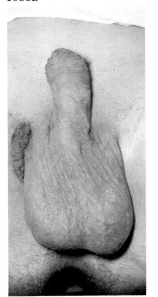

1088b

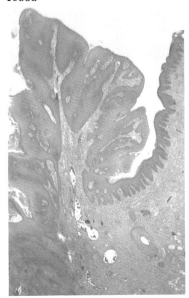

1089　Epithelial cysts of scrotal skin are common and a small typical cyst is shown.

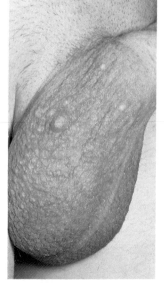

1089

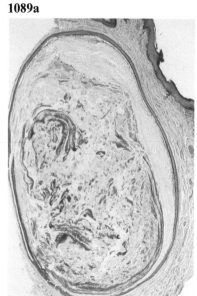

1089a

1089a　Section of a small cyst filled with keratin. Sometimes they rupture and stimulate a foreign body giant cell reaction in the surrounding tissue. Sometimes only cyst contents remain, with little or no reaction. *(H&E × 16)*

1090 and 1091　Oil cancers of the scrotum are a now rare form of occupational cancer, sometimes presenting in workers in the engineering and textile industries. An early and late form are shown. The histological pattern is no different to any squamous-cell skin carcinoma despite the chemical aetiology.

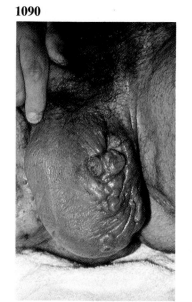

1090

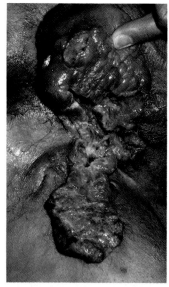

1091

1092　Other scrotal tumours are rare and a spindle-cell sarcoma is shown.

1093　Scrotum:　spindle-cell　sarcoma. Sections show that the tumour is made up of sheets of poorly differentiated cells which are elongated. Mitoses are prominent. *(H&E × 256)*

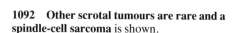

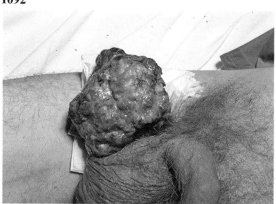

1092

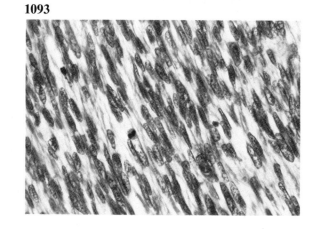

1093

12   Diseases of the testis

Enlargement of the scrotal contents are of great clinical importance because of the difficulties with differential diagnosis and the necessity for early confirmation of testicular tumour. Simple painless enlargements are usually found to be cystic. Hydroceles are normally primary (idiopathic), transilluminated brilliantly and unless very lax the testis cannot be palpated. Secondary hydroceles are associated with testicular pathology.

1094   A hydrocele enlarges the scrotum and unlike an inguinal hernia the upper extent of the swelling can be easily determined.

1094

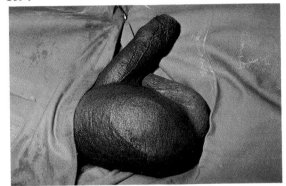

1095

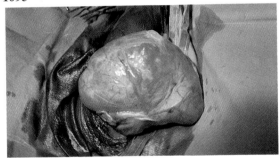

1095   When the scrotal skin is reflected the hydrocele and its covering are displayed.

1096

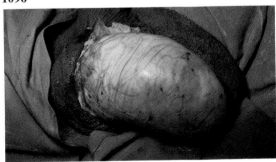

1096   Further dissection displays the thin wall of the hydrocele sac.

1097

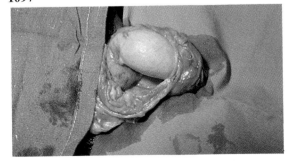

1097   When the sac is opened the normal testis is visible.

1098

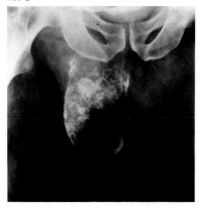

1099

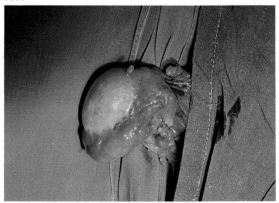

1098 In very longstanding hydroceles a rare complication of calcification of the wall may occur. Usually this is post-traumatic.

Appendix testis

1099 A testicular appendage, the hydatid of Morgagni, can be seen at the upper pole. These appendages can undergo torsion.

1100 These appendages may be bilateral.

1100

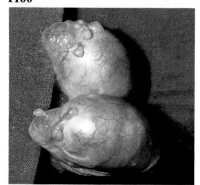

1101 This vestigial structure (also called the hydatid of Morgagni) is derived from the upper end of the paramesonephric duct. It is composed of a core of vascular connective tissue and is normally covered by columnar or cuboidal epithelium. *(H&E × 26)*

1101

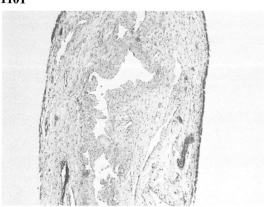

1102

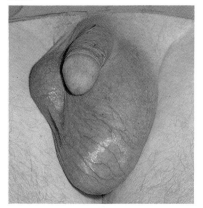

1102 The cyst of epididymis will usually have a similar scrotal contour to the hydrocele, but occasionally the testis may be observed below the cyst.

1103

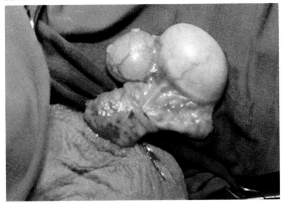

1104

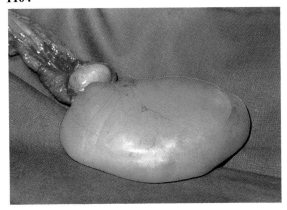

1103 Careful palpation will show that the testis can be palpated separately from the small cyst, here shown at exploration.

1104 A large epididymal cyst. Some contain spermatozoa and therefore can be termed spermatoceles. These tend to transilluminate less brilliantly than epididymal cysts and primary hydroceles.

1105

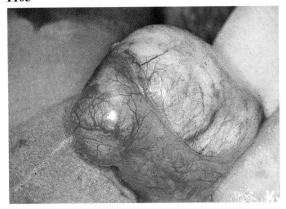

1105 This small epididymal cyst has arisen close to the body of the testis in the globus major.

1106

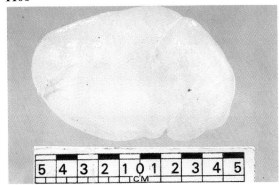

1106 Excised cyst of epididymis.

1107

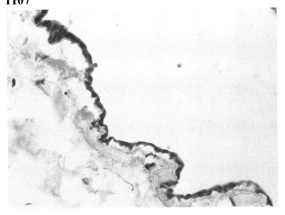

1107 Spermatoceles. These cysts contain sperm in the fluid but these are not seen in histological preparations. The epithelial lining is similar to a hydrocecle and is usually cuboidal, but this may be attenuated to form a flattened lining: occasionally a pseudostratified appearance is seen. There is loose connective tissue outside. *(H&E × 160)*

1108   Solid benign lesions may arise in the epididymis as painless swellings and cause difficulty with diagnosis.

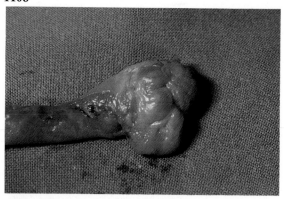

1109   Histology reveals a fibrous nodule which may have followed rupture of a cyst.

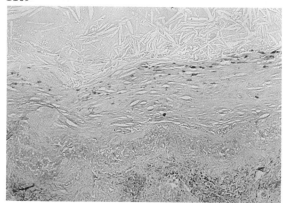

1110

Hydrocele fluid content
Clear
Specific gravity of more than 1020
Inorganic salts
Albumen
Fibrinogen
Cholesterol

1110 and 1111   The fluid aspirated from the cystic lesions of the scrotum differs according to the type of lesion.

1111

Epididymal cyst fluid content
Opalescent
Low specific gravity less than 1005
A small amount or no protein
Cells and occasional spermatozoa

1112

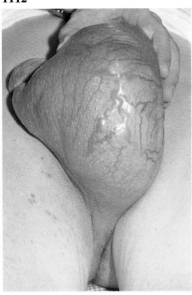

1113

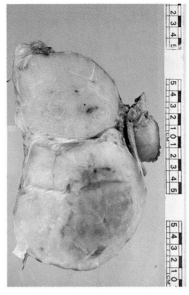

1114

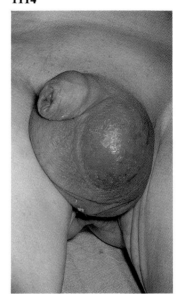

1112 Paratesticular lipoma. This massive tumour which felt lobulated, rubbery and did not transilluminate presenting in the scrotum and is causing congestion of the scrotal veins.

1113 Removal of the tumour and testis, to which it was closely adherent, revealed a large, lobulated, yellowish mass. Histology revealed mature adipose tissue with areas of fat necrosis. Despite the size of the mass there was no evidence of malignancy.

1114 Epididymitis. The enlarged inflamed epididymis and body of testis with associated scrotal erythema. A complication of urinary tract infection which can pose diagnostic problems as torsion may produce a similar clinical picture.

1115 Torsion. This lesion, which can rarely be bilateral, leads to a true urological emergency and may be very difficult to diagnose. In the infant, torsion of the whole cord may result in testicular infarction. In the adolescent, torsion of the body of the testis or of the body and epididymis occurs within the tunica vaginalis. In this condition the testis may lie horizontally, the so-called 'bell-clapper' testis. Diagnosis can be very difficult as the onset may not be dramatic and the pain initially not severe. When lying high in the scrotum the diagnosis may be easier to reach but this condition is very readily confused with epididymo-orchitis. If torsion is suspected, exploration is imperative as there are only six to eight hours from onset to irreversible infarction in most cases.

1116 The torted testis delivered at operation.

1115

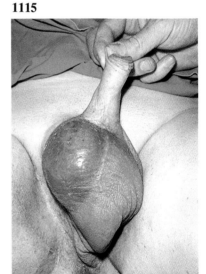

1116

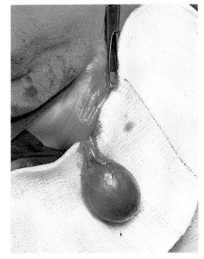

1117

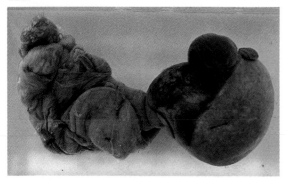

1118

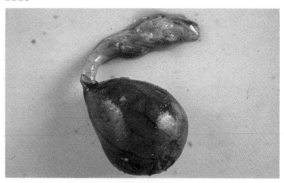

1119

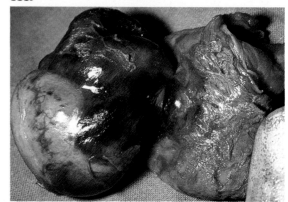

1120

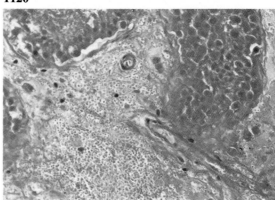

1121

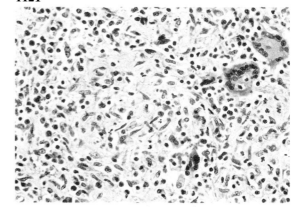

1117   Torsion: the whole cord is twisted here (formalin fixed).

1118   The resected specimen is seen to be infarcted (formalin fixed).

1119   The body of the testis is twisted within the tunica vaginalis and is deeply congested.

1120   This section shows the infarction which follows torsion. The ghost outlines of dead tubules are seen in the upper part of the field; haemorrhage is present in the oedematous loose connective tissue between. *(H&E × 50)*

1121   Granulomatous orchitis. Clinically presenting as a solid enlarged body of testis, this inflammatory lesion may be mistaken for a tumour both clinically and histologically. It is characterised by a chronic inflammatory-cell infiltration in which there are aggregates of histiocytes, some of which may be multinucleate. These granulomas are non-caseating and are thought to be a reaction to the contents of ruptured tubules. It is important to exclude tuberculosis. *(H&E × 160)*

1121a Varicocele. Classically the patient describes the feeling of a 'bag of worms' within his scrotum. These varicose veins transmit a cough impulse and arise from the pampiniform plexus, with or without a cremasteric element.

1121a

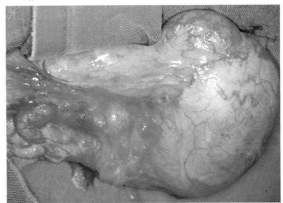

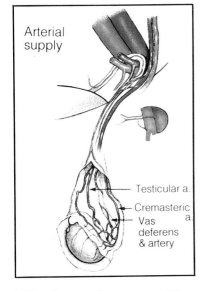

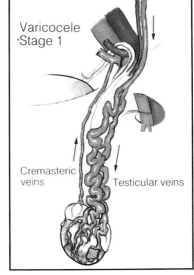

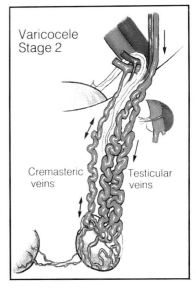

1122 The vascular anatomy of the cord.

1123 Stage I varicocele. The cremasteric veins are not involved.

1124 Stage II varicocele. The cremasteric veins are involved.

1125 Selective renal venography showing incompetence of the testicular vein valves.

1125a An enormous varicocele pushing up the ureter to the fundus of the bladder.

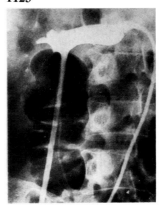

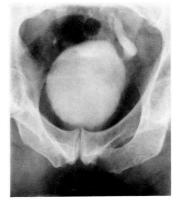

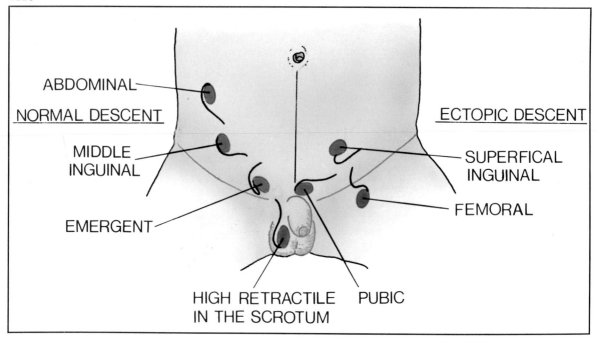

1126 Testicular maldescent. Diagram showing sites of incomplete and ectopic descent. Rarely penile and perineal ectopic testes are also found.

1127

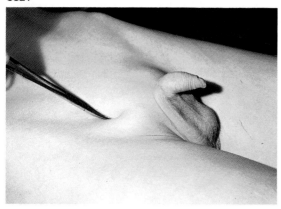

1128

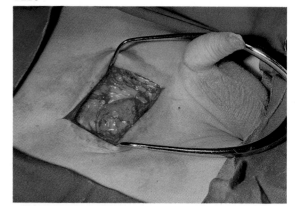

1127 The incompletely descended testis can be seen in the groin with the empty scrotum below.

1128 The inguinal testis displayed at exploration.

1129 The tubules in this specimen are lined by Sertoli cells and no spermatogenesis is apparent. The tubular basement membranes are hyalinised and there is peritubular fibrosis. Interstitial cells are prominent. *(H&E × 160)*

1129

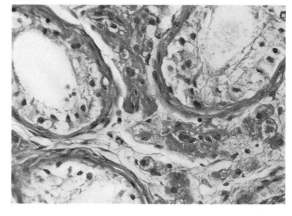

Testicular tumours

These tumours most commonly occur in men in their twenties and thirties. Although classically the tumour presents as an enlarging painless but heavy feeling testis, confusion often occurs in diagnosis because it has not been widely appreciated that more than one-third of the patients present with pain in the testis. Other presentations include the metastatic spread to the lungs and para-aortic nodes found at routine chest xray or on abdominal examination. It can also be an incidental finding during the investigation of infertility, either clinically or as an unsuspected lesion at testicular biopsy.

1130   At inspection the right testis is seen to be enlarged. The normal epididymis can normally be palpated. It is essential to differentiate between tumours and epididymo-orchitis, because both may present with pain. If a secondary hydrocele is present it is usually small.

Investigation is determined by the mode of spread by the lymphatics to the para-aortic nodes and the bloodstream to the lungs and other organs.

1130

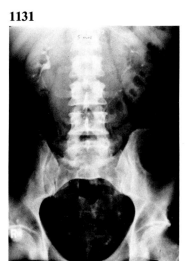

Investigations: testicular tumours

1 CXR with whole lung tomography if CT scanning not available.
2 Lymphangiography.
3 IVU.
4 CAT scanning.
5 Ultrasound of liver.

6 Blood markers –
   a) Serum alpha fetoprotein – normal range $1-10\,\mu g/1$.
   b) ß Human chorionic gonadotrophin – normal range $1-2\,\mu g/1$.
7 Liver function tests.
8 Renal function tests.
9 Full blood count.

1131

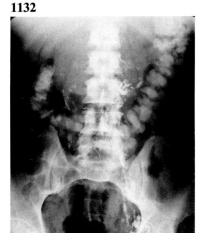

1132

1133

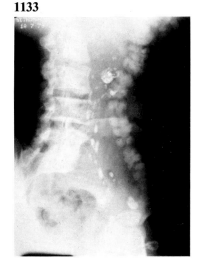

The specimens for the estimation of the markers must be taken before orchiectomy. Although the AFP is seldom raised in pure seminomas its elevation when a seminoma has been found in the resected specimen suggests that there is in fact a mixed tumour or the occasional situation of liver metastases from a pure seminoma. The AFP and ßHCG are frequently elevated in various types of teratoma. The AFP principally rises in the yolk sac tumour and the ßHCG in the chorion carcinoma. These markers will fall when all tumour is eradicated and are thus very valuable in demonstrating the presence of occult metastases which cannot be shown by other techniques. The importance of the normal plasma half-life of AFP at five days and ßHCG at 24–36 hours must be emphasised as the most significant method of assessing active disease, rather than their absolute values.

1131   IVU. The kidneys may be displaced laterally and rotated outwards by a para ortic mass of glands as shown here.

1132 and 1133 Lymphangiography will confirm enlarged and abnormal lymph nodes with metastases. The dye in the colon is from the IVU carried out before the lymphogram. A lateral view is also shown.

1134

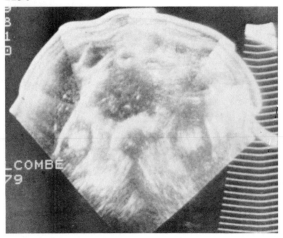

1135

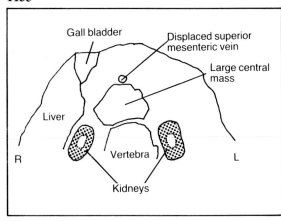

1134, 1135, 1136 and 1137   Ultrasound confirms the presence of a large para-aortic mass of glands in both transverse and longitudinal views.

1136

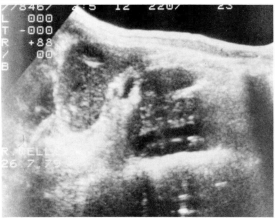

1137

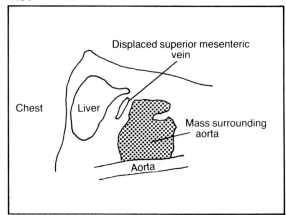

1138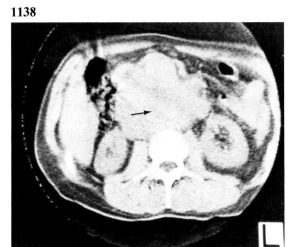

1139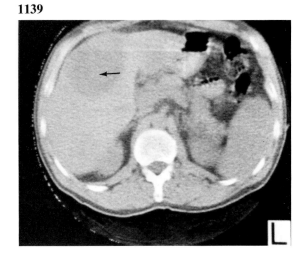

1138 CAT scans confirm the presence of a vast mass of metastatic para-aortic nodes (arrowed).

1139 The liver may be involved and the CAT scan here shows liver metastases from a seminoma (arrowed).

1140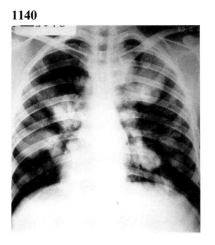

1141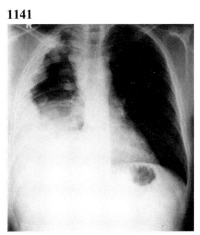

1142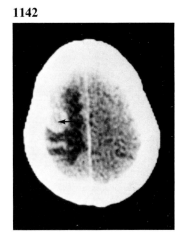

1140 Pulmonary metastases may be the presenting sign of testicular tumours.

1141 Gross metastatic pulmonary disease may result from progression of the condition with pleural involvement.

1142 Cerebral metastases may also be found and confirmed here by CAT scan. Unilateral neurological symptoms and signs should alert the clinician to this possibility (arrowed).

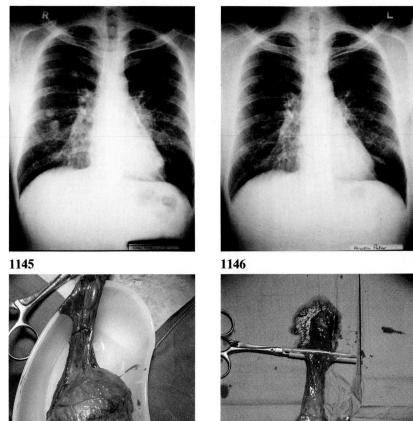

1143 Spontaneous regression of pulmonary metastases in testicular tumour is rare but recognised, following removal of the primary tumour. Multiple secondaries are seen in the lung fields.

1144 In this patient further pulmonary metastases developed subsequently. But here the lung fields have cleared following orchiectomy alone.

1145 The diagnosis is only proved by exploration. The groin is explored and the cord occluded with a non-crushing clamp. This expanded testis with its engorged veins is obviously grossly pathological.

1146 The excised testis is bisected and the tumour displayed.

1147

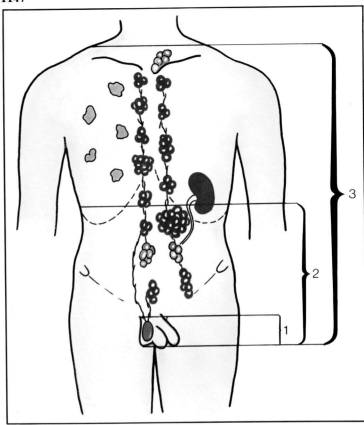

1147 Clinical staging of testicular tumours.
Stage 1 The tumour is confined to the testis.
Stage 2 There is involvement of the abdominal lymph nodes which are either manually palpable or demonstrated by radiological or other investigations.
Stage 3 Widespread metastases are present.

Primary tumours of the testis

Classification of testicular tumours is difficult because the conventional basis of histological typing, namely the cell of origin of the tumour, is hard to define when dealing with tumours which differentiate along many different lines. The main problem occurs with the definition of 'teratoma' and which tumours to include in this group.

Seminoma	Typical (well or poorly differentiated)
	Spermatocytic
Teratoma	Differentiated
	Intermediate
	Undifferentiated
	Trophoblastic

Combined seminoma and teratoma
Yolk sac tumour
Others: including interstitial cell tumour, Sertoli-cell tumour, gonadoblastoma, lymphoma, connective-tissue tumours.

Nomenclature of germ-cell tumours

The nomenclature of tumours which are believed to arise from testicular germ cells is not universally agreed. Most classifications distinguish seminoma and its subtypes from the others. Significant differences occur in the labelling of the non-seminoma group.

British classifications group the non-seminomas together as teratomas and distinguish them on the basis of:
1 Embryonic or extra embryonic differentiation (the latter includes trophoblastic and yolk-sac elements);
2 The degree of differentiation of the embryonic elements.

American nomenclature reserves the term 'teratoma' for those tumours containing recognisable tissue of more than one germ layer. Less well-differentiated tumours which nevertheless have a poorly differentiated epithelial or embryonic appearance are called 'embryonal carcinoma'. Tumours with trophoblastic differentiation are named 'choriocarcinoma', whether or not other elements are present. (See Table 8 – appendix)

The so-called orchioblastoma (or adenocarcinoma of the infant testis) is now recognised as yolk-sac differentiation of a germ-cell tumour. This pattern of differentiation is more and more frequently recognised in adult germ-cell tumours.

1148

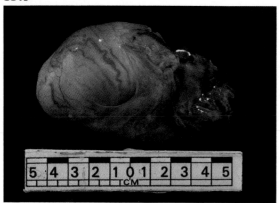

1149

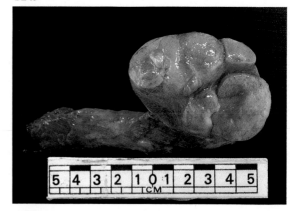

1148 Seminoma. Orchidectomy specimen. An enlarged testis but with no evidence of invasion through the tunica vaginalis.

1149 Seminoma. Cut surface of the specimen seen in **1148**. This tumour is slightly lobulated with a fairly homogeneous appearance. In the upper pole there is a yellowish area which is an area of infarction, often seen in seminomas. These tumours may be bilateral.

1150 Seminoma: well differentiated (typical). The tumour is composed of sheets of cells with delicate cytoplasm with large round nuclei and prominent nucleoli. There are scattered lymphocytes in the background and fine connective tissue bands often run between the tumour cells. *(H&E × 160)*

1150

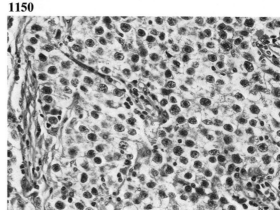

1151 Seminoma: well differentiated (typical). Higher magnification of the tumour seen in **1150**. The tumour cells are fairly regular and mitoses are infrequent (none in this field). Though the cytoplasm is delicate the cell boundaries are well seen. *(H&E × 256)*

1151

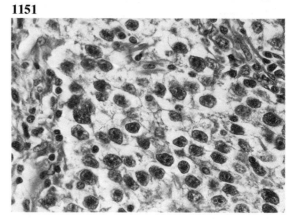

1152 Seminoma: (poorly differentiated). This tumour is similar to the typical seminoma on naked-eye examination, but microscopically it is different. Most important is the prominence of mitoses (five are present in this field), and there is also greater irregularity in the nuclei. The prognosis of these tumours is worse than for well differentiated seminomas. These are sometimes called anaplastic seminomas. *(H&E × 256)*

1152

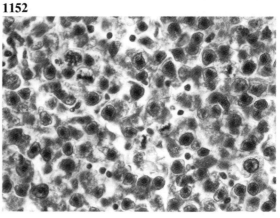

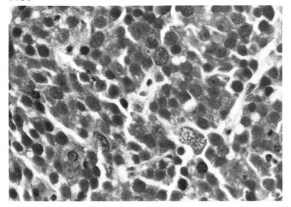

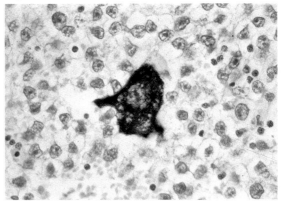

1153 Seminoma: spermatocytic. This tumour is distinguished from typical seminoma because of its histological appearances and better prognosis. Most of the cells are regular and have a round nucleus and eosinophilic cytoplasm. Other cells resemble secondary spermatocytes. A third type is a very large cell. *(H&E × 256)*

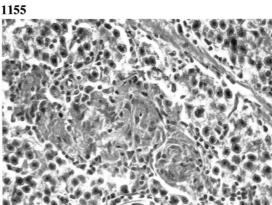

1154 Seminoma: syncytial giant cells. Multinucleate giant cells, resembling syncytial trophoblast are occasionally seen in seminomas. By immunohistology they can be shown to contain HCG (human chorionic gonadotrophin). At the moment their significance is not known. *(Immunoperoxidase for β subunit of HCG. × 160)*

1155 Seminoma: granulomatous reaction. This section shows a seminoma, but in the centre of the field is a collection of large cells with plentiful eosinophilic cytoplasm, some of which are multinucleate. This is a giant-cell granuloma, a similar lesion to that seen in inflammatory conditions such as sarcoidosis. Lymphocytic infiltration and granulomata are thought to be host responses to the presence of the tumour. *(H&E × 160)*

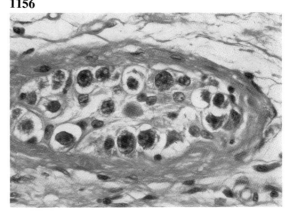

1156 Seminoma: dysplastic cells in adjacent tubule. This is an abnormal tubule filled with highly atypical cells. It is close to a seminoma. It may represent invasion of the seminoma along the tubule but there are claims that such lesions represent in situ malignant change which occurs before the development of invasive germ-cell tumours. *(H&E × 256)*

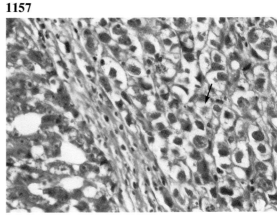

1157 Combined seminoma and teratoma. The right side of the field shows a tumour with the appearances of a seminoma (arrowed), the left side shows a teratoma. Where such combinations occur the tumour has the prognosis of the teratoma. *(H&E × 160)*

1158

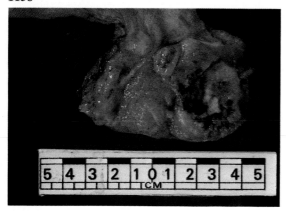

1159

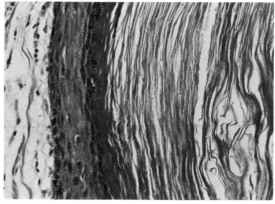

1158 Teratoma. Section through a testis containing a tumour showing widespread areas of haemorrhage and necrosis.

1159 Teratoma differentiated (WHO equivalent: teratoma mature or immature). Part of a tumour showing differentiation along many cell lines all of them being well-differentiated tissue with no evidence of malignancy. This area shows a well-differentiated stratified squamous epithelium which is keratinising. Though all elements appear benign the behaviour of some of these tumours is malignant. *(H&E × 160)*

1160 Teratoma differentiated (WHO equivalent: teratoma mature or immature). Another area of the tumour shown in **1159**, but this shows a well-differentiated mucus-secreting epithelium. In children this type of tumour may contain immature elements which do not imply malignancy. *(H&E × 160)*

1161 Teratoma: intermediate (WHO equivalent: embryonal carcinoma and teratoma with malignant transformation). A malignant teratoma containing incompletely differentiated tissue and cells having the features of malignancy. This section shows cuboidal epithelium in the top right corner; there is poorly formed cartilage in the bottom left corner and incompletely differentiated tissue between. *(H&E × 64)*

1160

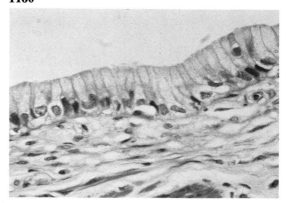

1161

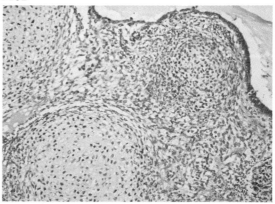

1162

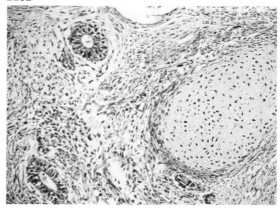

1162 Malignant teratoma intermediate (WHO equivalent: embryonal carcinoma and teratoma or teratoma with malignant transformation). Similar to **1161** with cartilage, glands and undifferentiated tissue. *(H&E × 64)*

1163

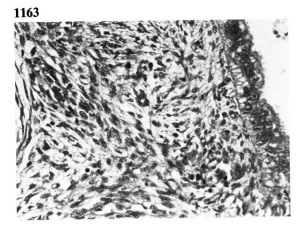

1164

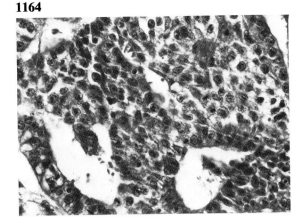

1163 Malignant teratoma intermediate (WHO equivalent: embryonal carcinoma and teratoma or teratoma with malignant transformation). Higher magnification showing an epithelium with cellular atypicality and stroma with mitotic figures. *(H&E × 160)*

1164 Malignant teratoma undifferentiated (WHO equivalent: embryonal carcinoma). A malignant teratoma lacking mature elements but which has a variable appearance, often with some differentiation suggesting an adenocarcinoma. *(H&E × 256)*

1165 Malignant teratoma trophoblastic. This testis shows a haemorrhagic mass at one pole. This was composed predominantly of trophoblastic tissue.

1165

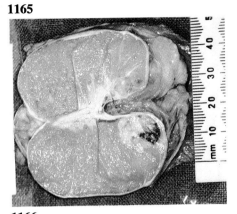

1166

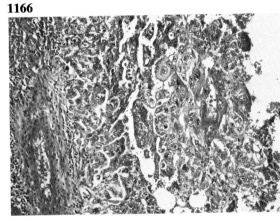

1166 Malignant teratoma trophoblastic (WHO equivalent: choriocarcinoma alone or with embryonal carcinoma or other germ-cell tumour). A malignant teratoma with extra embryonic differentiation to trophoblast. The section shows cyto and syncytio-trophoblast arranged in a villous pattern. *(H&E × 64)*

1167

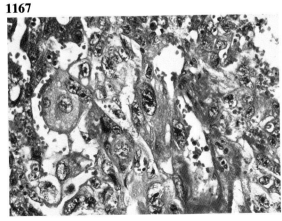

1167 Malignant teratoma trophoblastic. A higher magnification of the specimen in **1166** to show syncytiotrophoblast. Trophoblastic differentiation in a teratoma carries a worse prognosis. *(H&E × 256)*

1168

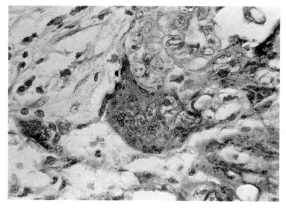

1169

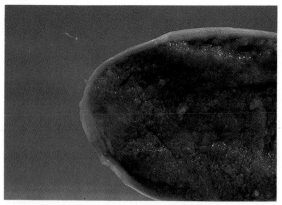

1170

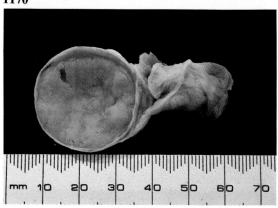

1171

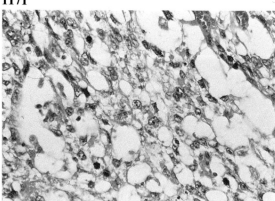

1172

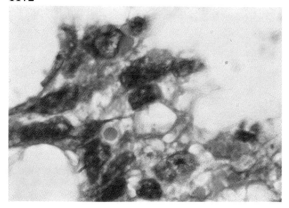

1168 Malignant teratoma trophoblastic. This type of tumour was one of the first to be associated with a 'tumour marker' detectable in the serum or urine, human chorionic gonadotrophin (HCG). The hormone produced by the tumour cells may also be demonstrated in the tissue by the use of labelled antiserum to the tumour product. In this section HCG has been demonstrated by using antiserum to its ß subunit to localise an enzyme, a peroxidase, to the HCG containing cells: the peroxidase produces a brown reaction product from a substrate. The brown stain represents sites where HCG is present. *(Immuno-peroxidase immunocytochemistry for HCG × 256)*

1169 Malignant teratoma. Occasionally a primary tumour may scar up while metastases kill the patient. This testis comes from a patient who died with wide-spread metastases of a malignant teratoma. The only lesion seen in either testis was this scar at one pole of the left testis.

1170 Yolk-sac tumour (synonyms include: orchio-blastoma, endodermal sinus tumour, adenocarcinoma of the infant testis). Pure yolk-sac tumour tend to occur in infants. This is one in a child of nine months. The cut surface shows a well circumscribed yellowish tumour. Yolk-sac elements may be found in adult teratomas and tend to be associated with a poorer prognosis: like trophoblastic elements, they represent extra-embryonic development of a teratoma.

1171 Yolk-sac tumour (orchioblastoma). The tumour typically grows in a pattern of a loose vacuolated network with apparent glandular differentiation which gave rise to its designation as 'adenocarcinoma'. *(H&E × 160)*

1172 Yolk-sac tumour. A higher magnification shows the eosinophilic globules in the cytoplasm of cells. The globules can be shown to contain ∝ fetoprotein, an oncofoetal antigen which may also be present in the serum of patients with this tumour.

1173

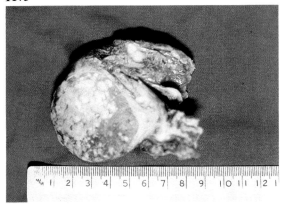

1174

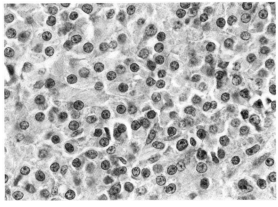

1175

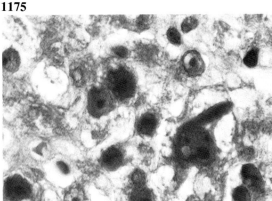

1176

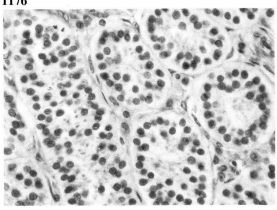

1177

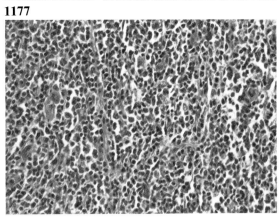

1173 Interstitial-cell tumour (Leydig-cell tumour). These tumours are yellow to brown on naked-eye examination; they measure up to 10 cm in diameter and are often lobulated. They may be hormonally active, tending to give virilisation in childhood and feminisation in adults. Most are benign but about 10 per cent metastasise.

1174 Interstitial-cell tumour (Leydig-cell tumour). The tumour consists of regular polygonal cells with eosinophilic or vacuolated cytoplasm. The nuclei are round to oval and contain small nucleoli. Large cells which are sometimes binucleate or multinucleate are occasionally present. *(H&E × 256)*

1175 Interstitial-cell tumour: Reinke crystalloids. These cytoplasmic inclusions are a marker of interstitial cells. They are rod-shaped structures that are difficult to see with haematoxylin and eosin, but more easily demonstrated with Masson's trichrome. They are seen in less than half of interstitial-cell tumours. *(Masson trichrome × 640)*

1176 Sertoli-cell tumour. This specimen shows a well differentiated Sertoli-cell tumour with clear cells arranged in a tubular fashion; less well-differentiated tumours cause diagnostic problems. Their behaviour is usually benign but metastasis can occur. *(H&E × 256)*

1177 Testis: malignant lymphoma. The testis may be the site of a primary malignant lymphoma or it may be secondarily involved in a generalised lymphoma. It tends to occur in older patients. This tumour shows sheets of small darkly staining cells with little cytoplasm. This is a lymphosarcoma. *(H&E × 160)*

1178   Adenomatoid tumour. This is the commonest tumour of paratesticular tissues and is benign. They are small, usually asymptomatic nodules. This section shows that it is composed of gland-like structures and stroma. *(H&E × 160)*

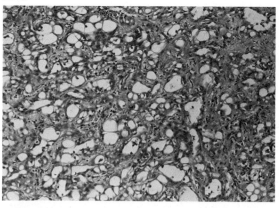

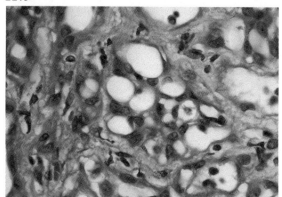

1179   Adenomatoid tumour. A higher magnification of the tumour in picture **1178** showing the characteristic mixture of connective tissue and spaces lined by flattened or cuboidal cells, some of which are vacuolated. The term 'mesothelioma' is sometimes loosely applied to these lesions. True mesothelioma may rarely occur in the tunica vaginalis and is a malignant tumour, more often seen in pleura and peritoneum. *(H&E × 256)*

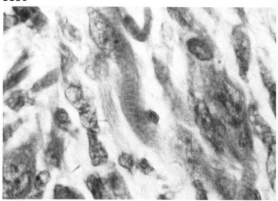

1180   Paratesticular rhabdomyosarcoma. Although it is rare, this tumour is relatively common among paratesticular malignancies. The histological pattern varies, but this section shows strap-like cells with pleomorphic nuclei and cross-striations in the cytoplasm of some cells. *(H&E × 640)*

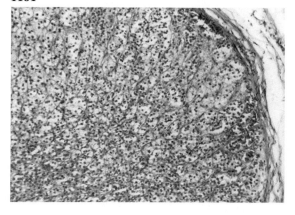

1181   Spermatic cord: adrenal rest. These developmental abnormalities may occur in the spermatic cord or in the rete testis. The arrangement of cells resembles that of the zona fasciculata in the adrenal cortex. They are quite benign. *(H&E × 64)*

Testicular tubule morphology

Illustration of the many lesions seen in the testes of the subfertile male is beyond the scope of this work, but some of the commoner lesions are illustrated below. In biopsy of the testis for an assessment of morphology formol saline is an inadequate fixative because it causes considerable distortion and poor preservation. Bouin's fluid gives much better preservation.

Testis: normal

1182 and 1183   Testicular tubules with Sertoli cells and germ cells with maturation through spermatocytes and spermatids to spermatozoa (in the centre of the tubule). The basement membrane and associated connective tissue is of normal size. The intertubular connective tissue is loose and interstitial cells are not prominent.

1182   *(H&E × 160)*

1183   *(H&E × 256)*

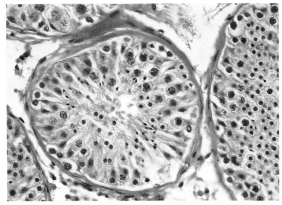

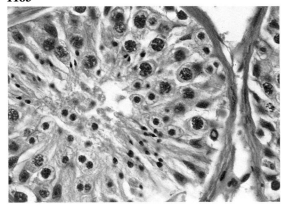

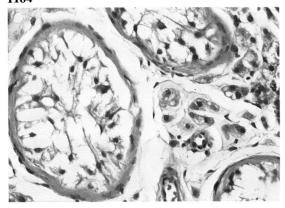

1184   Undescended testis. The tubules in this specimen are lined by Sertoli cells and no spermiogenesis is apparent. The tubular basement membranes are hyalinised and there is peritubular fibrosis. Interstitial cells are prominent. *(H&E × 160)*

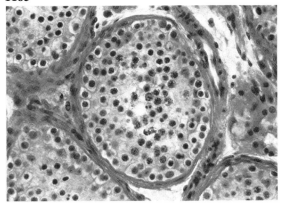

1185   Testis: maturation arrest. In this abnormality maturation of spermatozoa is halted and failure of spermatogenesis results. These tubules show Sertoli cells, germ cells and spermatocytes but virtually nothing beyond that. *(H&E × 160)*

1186 Testis: Klinefelter's syndrome. This biopsy (from a chromatin positive Klinefelter's syndrome) shows tubules lined with Sertoli cells, hyalinised basement membranes and no spermiogenesis. There are very prominent masses of interstitial cells. *(H&E × 160)*

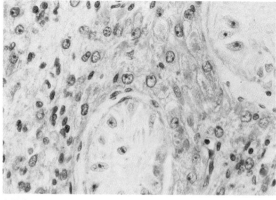

1187 Testis: post-mumps orchitis. This biopsy came from a subfertile patient with a history of mumps orchitis. There were patchy lesions in the testis where, as illustrated by this section, tubules showed atrophy of lining cells, marked hyalinisation of the basement membrane and fibrosis of the interstitial tissue. *(H&E × 160)*

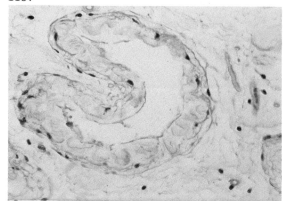

1188 Testis: testicular feminisation. This term refers to the syndrome of a genetic male with a female body form and external genitalia but with no uterus or tubes and little axillary and pubic hair. The testis is composed of small tubules with no spermiogenesis; they are immature and similar to those in the prepubertal male. The interstitial cells are very prominent. *(H&E × 160)*

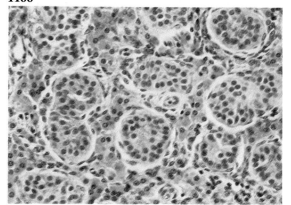

Appendix

Microbiology

Urinanalysis

Mid-stream specimen – MSU. In males a correctly taken mid-stream specimen will give high correalation with bladder urine, except where acute prostatic or urethral infection exists.

Clean-catch specimen – CCSU. In females urethral contaminant bacteria may obscure the exact status of infection in the urinary tract, especially when low counts of bacteria are present.

Suprapubic aspiration – SPA. Urine obtained by this technique will show precisely whether or not there is bacterial infection of bladder urine, and is particularly useful in women and neonates.

Upper-tract localisation – UTL. Segregated specimens of urine taken cystoscopically during diuresis will identify precisely the site of infection in the upper tracts.

Lower-tract localisation – LTL. Similar studies of the lower tract can distinguish between urethral, prostatic or vesical urinary infection.

Early-morning specimens of urine – EMU. Early-morning specimens of urine are used to isolate myco-bacterium. Three or preferably five consecutive specimens are inoculated on to artificial culture media with and without pyruvate. Animal inoculation tests are now very rarely required.

(Tables 1 to 4 relate to Chapter 1)

Table 1. Normal urine values of interest to the urologist.

Specific gravity	1.015–1.030	
pH	6.5–7.5	
Sodium	100–250 mmol/24 hr	8–15 g/24 hr
Potassium	30–90 mmol/24 hr	1.4–3.5 g/24 hr
Chlorides	150–200 mmol/24 hr	3.5–4.0 g/24 hr
Calcium	2.5–7.5 mmol/24 hr F	100–300 mg/24 hr M
	2.5–9 mmol/24 hr M	100–360 mg/24 hr F
Phosphate	15–50 mmol/24 hr	0.5–1.5 g/24 hr
Urate	3.12 mmol/24 hr	0.5–20 mg/24 hr
Oxalates	0.11–0.66 mmol/24 hr	15–20 mg/24 hr
Magnesium	7.0–12.5 mmol/24 hr	0.17–0.29 g/24 hr
Urea	160–600 mmol/24 hr	10–35 g/24 hr
Creatinine	13–18 mmol/24 hr	1.5–2.0 g/24 hr M
	7–13 mmol/24 hr	0.8–1.5 g/24 hr F
Catecholamines	less than 0.55 mol/24 hr	less than 100 g/24 hr
Hydroxymethoxymandelate		
HMMA	range 0.7–2.5 μg per mg creatinine	
17 Oxosteroids	as dehydrodepiandrosterone	
17 Oxogenic steroids		
17 Oxosteroids	20–85 μmol/24 hr M	3–23 mg/24 hr M
	14–70 μmol/24 hr F	2–20 mg/24 hr F
17 Hydroxycortico steroids	25–70 μmol/24 hr M	5–20 mg/24 hr M
	16–65 μmol/24 hr F	4–17 mg/24 hr F
Hydroxyprolin	0.1–0.6 mmol/g creatinine/24 hr	6–40 mg/g creatinine/24 hr
Renal function tests		
creatinine clearance	90–130 ml/mm	
PSP 1st half hour	50–60 per cent recovery	
2nd half hour	10–15 per cent recovery	

Table 2. Normal seminal analysis.

Volume	2–6 ml
Viscosity	Complete liquifaction 45 minutes after ejaculation
Sperm density	20–200 10^6/ml
Total number of spermatazoa per ejaculate	>80 10^6
Live spermatazoa	>60 per cent
Motile spermatazoa progressive	>60 per cent
Normal spermatazoa	>70 per cent
Fructose	8–25 mmol/l
Citric acid	250–800 mg/100 ml
Zinc	1.5–4 mmol/l
Magnesium	3–10 mmol/l
Acid phosphatase	250–500 10×10^{-2}/ml
Glyceryl phosphoryl choline	110–150 mg per cent
Carnitine	400–500 μmol/l

Table 3. Normal haematological values.

Red blood cells	$4-6\,10^{12}/l$
White blood cells	$4-10\,10^{9}/l$
Haemoglobin	12–17 g/dl
PCV	0.35–0.5
MCV	76–96 fl
MCH	29–32 pg
McHC	32–36 g/dl
Platelets	150–500 thousand
Reticulocytes	1–2 per cent
Differential	
Neutrophils	50–65 per cent
Lymphocytes	30–45 per cent
Monocytes	10–12 per cent
Eosinophils	1–3 per cent
Basophils	1–7 per cent
ESR	1–7 mm in the first hour

Table 4. Normal blood chemical values of interest to the urologist.

p – plasma, s – serum

Sodium p	135–145 mmol/l	
Chlorides p	95–105 mmol/l	
Potassium p	3.5–5.0 mmol/l	
Bicarbonate p	22–28 mmol/l	
Calcium s	2.2–2.6 mmol/l	8.8–10.4 mg/100 ml
Phosphate p	0.8–1.4 mmol/l	2.5–5.4 mg/100 ml
Magnesium p	0.7–1.1 mmol/l	1.6–2.7 mg/100 ml
Creatinine s	60–100 μmol/l	0.7–1.1 mg/100 ml
Urea p	2.5–6.5 mmol/l	15–40 mg/100 ml
Uric acid s	150–400 μmol/l F	2.5–6.7 mg/100 ml
	150–500 μmol/l M	2.5–8.4 mg/100 ml
Glucose s	3.3–5.0 mmol/l	60–90 mg/100 ml
Albumin s	45–50 g/l	
Globulin s	15–30 g/l total 60–80 g/l	
Fibrinogen p	2–4 g/l	
Immunoglobulins		
IGA	80–200 IU/ml	150–350 mg/100 ml
IGG	90–180 IU/ml	800–1500 mg/100 ml
IGM	90–210 IU/ml	80–180 mg/100 ml
Alpha-fetoprotein (ADP) s		0–30 mg/ml
Bilirubin s	5–17 μmol/l	0.4–1 mg/100 ml
Alkaline phosphatase s	20–90 IU/l	3–30 King-Armstrong units/100 ml
Alanine (GPT)		
Transaminase (ALT)	5–40 IU/l	
Aspartate (GOT)		
Transaminase (ASP) s	10–40 IU/l	
Lactate dehydroginase		
(LDH) s	50–225 IU/l	200–680 units/ml serum
Acid phosphatase s	total up to 11 IU/l	0.5–4.0 King-Armstrong units/100 ml
	formol stable up to 4 IU/l	0.–0.5 King-Armstrong units/100 ml
Cholesterol s	3.6–7.8 mmol/l	40–290 mg/100 ml
ß Lipoproteins s	3.5 g/l	
Triglyceride mephalometry		
(as Triolein) s	0.25–1.80 g/l	
LH cortisol p	200–700 mmol/l	7.2–25.8 μg/100 ml

(Tables 5 and 6 are related to Chapter 9)

Table 5 UICC (TNM).   Classification as applied to prostatic tumours.

Tx   Incidental carcinoma in operative specimen: i.e. no pre-operative evidence of carcinoma or where the carcinoma was previously unsuspected. This will be linked with a P category in operative specimen.

T1   Intracapsular malignancy involving less than 50 per cent total volume of prostate in an otherwise normal or hypertrophied gland – the nodule.

T2   Intracapsular malignancy involving more than 50 per cent of the volume of an otherwise normal or hypertrophic gland.

T3   Malignancy extending beyond capsule into the para-prostatic tissue. This includes cases with involvement of seminal vesicle, ulceration in posterior urethra, or invasion of bladder-neck.

T4   Malignancy fixed to pelvic wall and/or involvement of rectum and/or bladder beyond bladder-neck.

To   No evidence of primary growth but clinical diagnosis of metastatic prostatic cancer made. (Will be linked with N2 or M1 category.)

Tis   Pre-invasive carcinoma (carcinoma in situ)

Px   Pathologist is not able to give extent of the tumour, but did have malignant tissue available for examination – as in casual TUR.

P1   Malignant intracapsular nodule occupying less than 50 per cent volume of the whole prostate.

P2   Malignant change involving more than 50 per cent volume of the prostate.

P3   Involvement of capsule or incomplete removal of malignancy.

G   Histopathological grading.

G1   High degree of differentiation.

G2   Medium degree of differentiation.

G3   Low degree of differentiation or undifferentiated.

GX   Grade cannot be assessed.

Table 6.   Prostate.

T0   Incidental carcinoma.

T1   Intracapsular/normal gland.

T2   Intracapsular/deformed gland.

T3   Extension beyond capsule.

T4   Extension fixed to neighbouring organs.

N1   Single homolateral regional.

N2   Contralateral or bilateral/multiple regional.

N3   Fixed regional.

N4   Juxtaregional.

M0   No metastases.

M1   Distant metastases.

MX   Not assessable.

(Table 7 is related to Chapter 11)

Table 7 Penis TNM.   Classification as applied to penile tumours.

Tis   Pre-invasive carcinoma (carcinoma in situ).

T0   No evidence of primary tumour.

T1   Tumour 2 cm or less in its largest dimension, strictly superficial or exophytic.

T2   Tumour more than 2 cm but less than 5 cm in its largest dimension or tumour with minimal extension.

T3   Tumour more than 5 cm in its largest dimension or tumour with deep extension, including the urethra.

T4   Tumour infiltrating neighbouring structures.

TX   The minimum requirements to assess the primary tumour cannot be met.

N   Regional lymph nodes.

N0   No evidence of regional lymph-node involvement.

N1   Evidence of involvement of movable unilateral regional lymph nodes.

N2   Evidence of involvement of movable bilateral regional lymph nodes.

N3   Evidence of involvement of fixed regional lymph nodes.

NX   Minimum requirements to assess the regional lymph nodes cannot be met.

M0   No metastases.

M1   Distant metastases.

MX   Not assessable.

(Table 8 is related to Chapter 12)

* **Table 8.   Equivalent terms in different teratoma classifications.**

Testicular tumour panel 1975	Armed Forces Institute of Pathology Fascicle 1973 (Mostofi & Price)	WHO 1975

Teratoma differentiated	Teratoma mature
	    immature
		Teratoma mature
		    immature

Malignant teratoma intermediate	Embryonal carcinoma with teratoma, with or without other elements	Teratoma with malignant transformation Embryonal carcinoma and teratoma

Malignant teratoma undifferentiated	Embryonal carcinoma
	    Adult
	    Infantile
	    Polyembryoma
		Embryonal carcinoma

Malignant teratoma trophoblastic	Choriocarcinoma with or without embryonal carcinoma	Choriocarcinoma with or without embryonal carcinoma or other germ-cell tumour

Pathology of the Testis, (Ed.) R.C.B. Pugh, Blackwell, 1976.

Index

All numbers indicate figure and caption numbers.

Appendix